Mariel's Kitchen

Mariel's Kitchen

Simple Ingredients for a Delicious and Satisfying Life

Mariel Hemingway

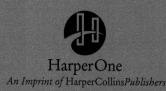

HarperOne
An Imprint of HarperCollinsPublishers

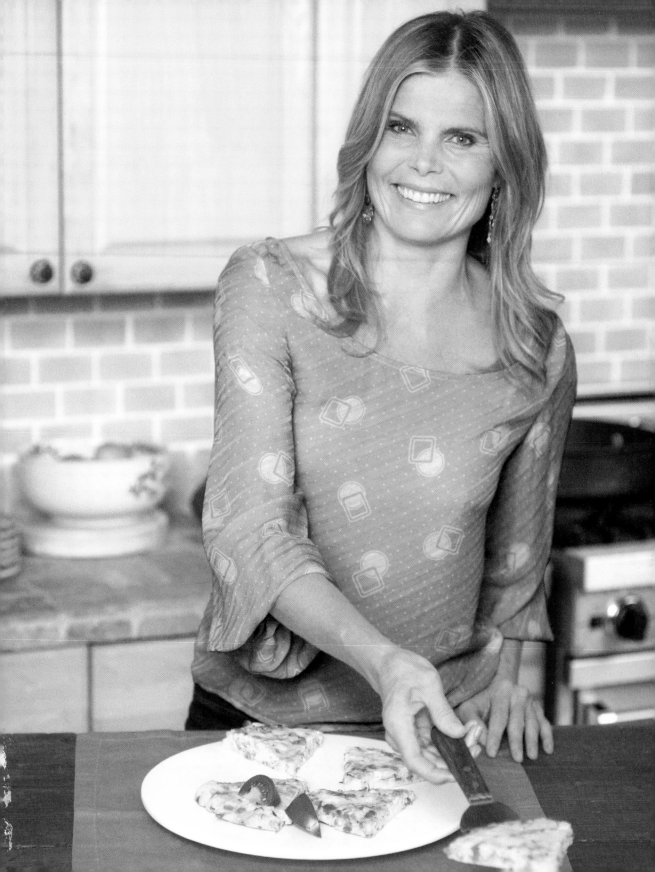

PHOTOGRAPHY

Photographer: Jeff Katz / JeffKatzPhotography.com

Associate Photographer: Andrew Strauss

Assistant Photographer: Stuart Gow

FOOD

Recipe Development: FoodFanatics.net

Food Styling: Denise Vivaldo and Cindie Flannigan
    of FoodFanatics.net

Assistant Food Stylist: Jennifer Park

Food Styling Interns: Sarah Bush and Travis Witten

Prop Designer: Matt Armendariz

Assistant Prop Designer: Karine Beaudry

WARDROBE AND PROPS

Wardrobe Mistress: Golriz Moeini

Clothing from: Magnolia, Calabasas, CA

Flowers by: Florentyna's, Calabasas, CA

BOOK PRODUCER

BTDNYC

Producer, Art Director, Designer: Beth Tondreau

Designer and Layout: Punyapol "Noom" Kittayarak

Associate Designer: Suzanne Dell'Orto

*Photos on pages: x bottom, xi bottom, xvi-xvii, xviii-xix, 7 bottom, 8 bottom, 25,
38, 43, 46, 108, 114, 116, 147, 152-153, 156, 157, 158 top, 159, 195,
196 top, 209, 210, 223, 228, 238, 254-255, 258 are by Beth Tondreau;
Photos on pages: 126 and 229 are by Punjapol "Noom" Kittayarak*

MARIEL'S KITCHEN

Simple Ingredients for a Delicious and Satisfying Life

FIRST EDITION

LIBRARY OF CONGRESS CATALOGING-IN-PUBLICATION DATA IS AVAILABLE.

ISBN: 978-0-06-164987-5

09 10 11 12 13   RRD(W)   10 9 8 7 6 5 4 3 2 1

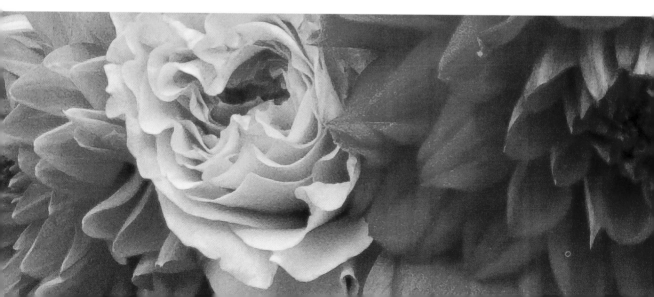

For my gorgeous girls

Dree Louise and Langley Fox

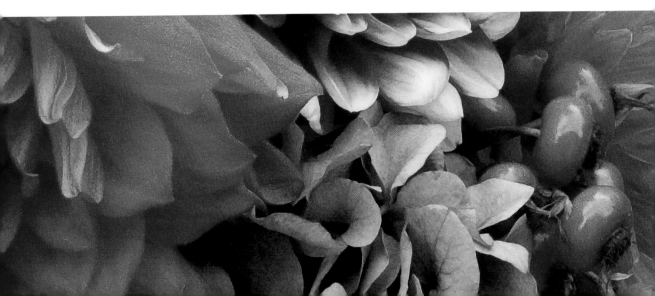

Contents

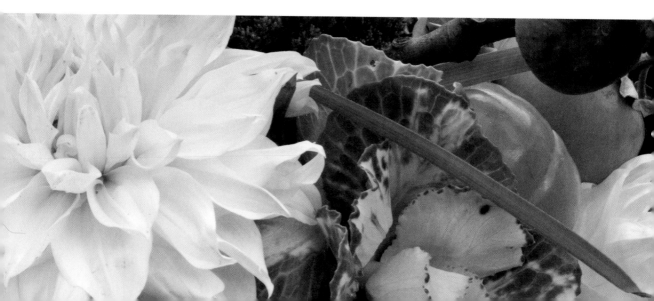

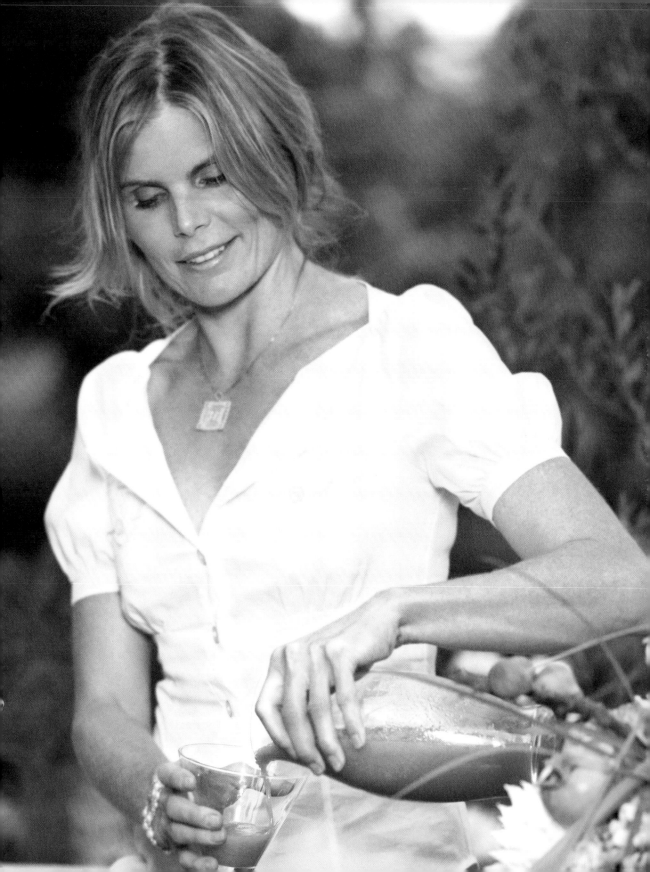

Essentials

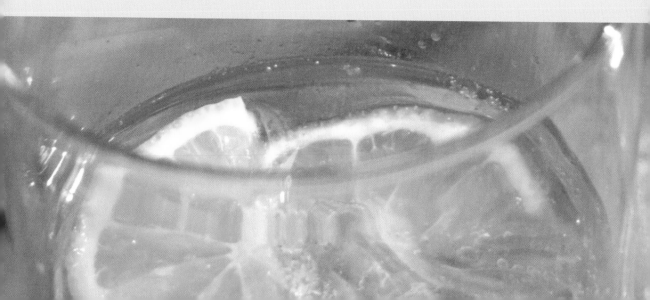

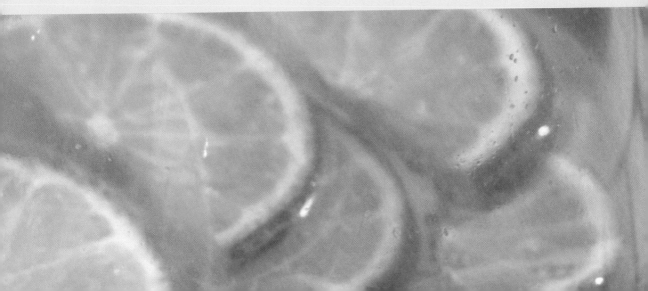

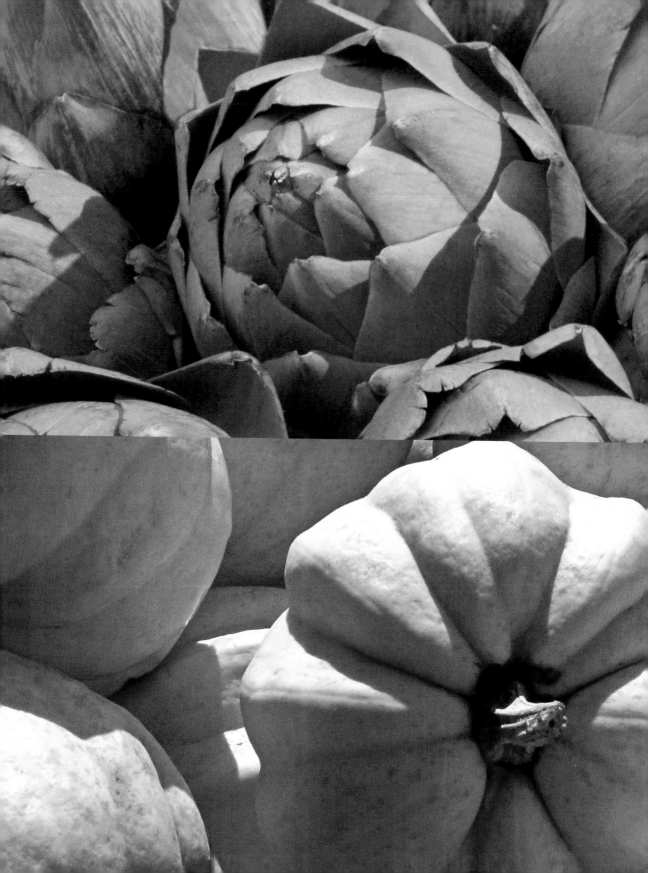

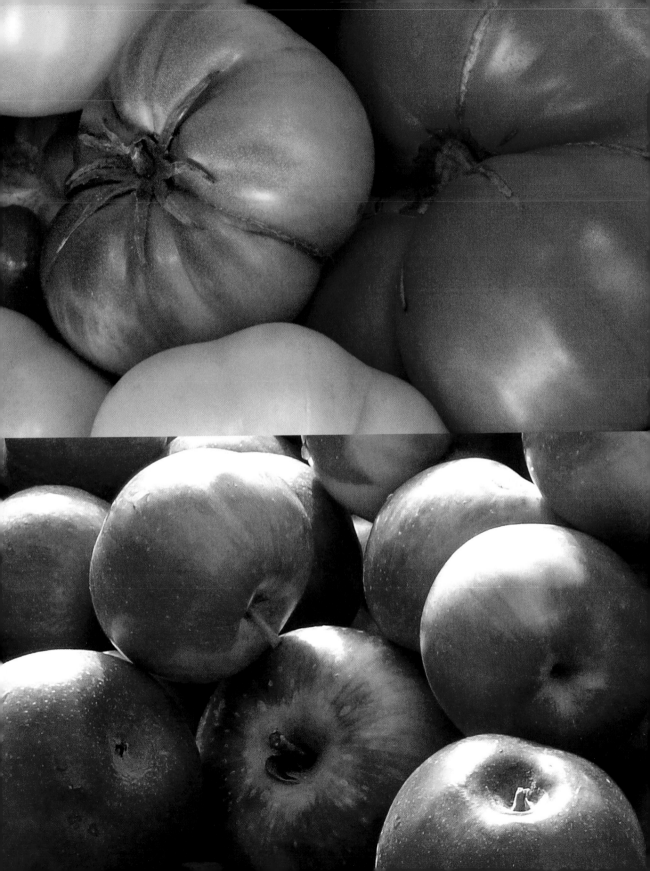

Spring

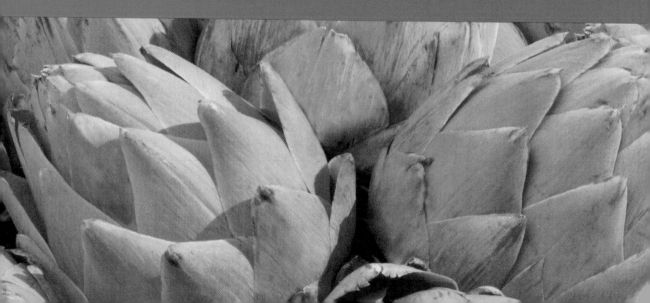

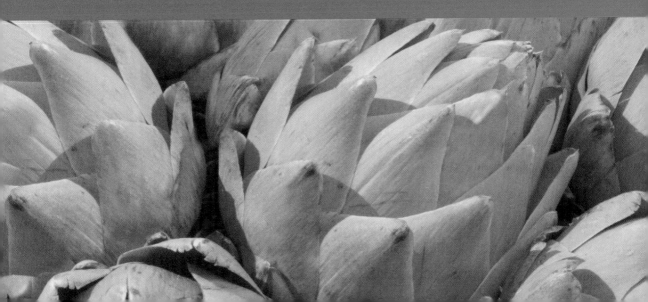

Summer

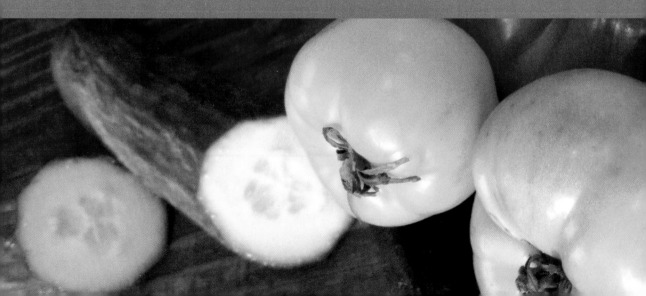

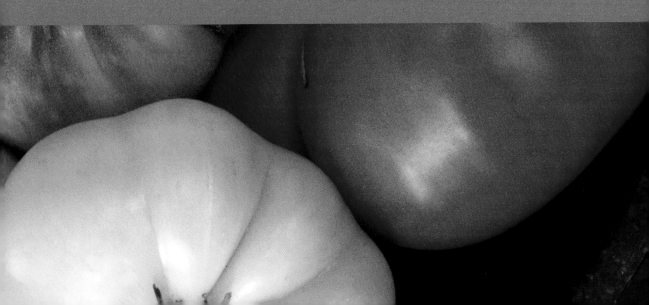

Fall

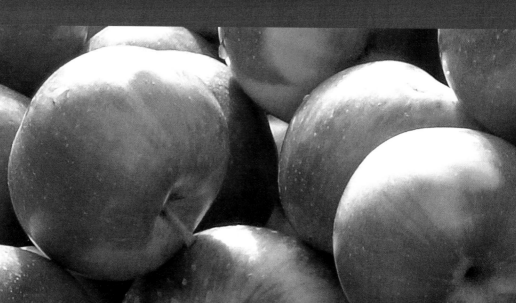

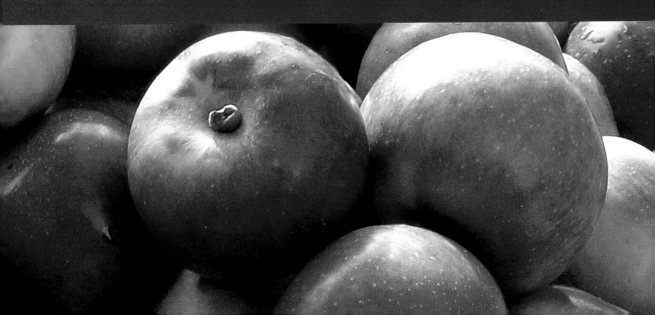

Winter

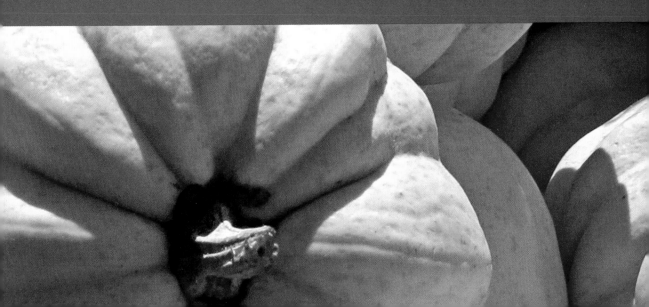

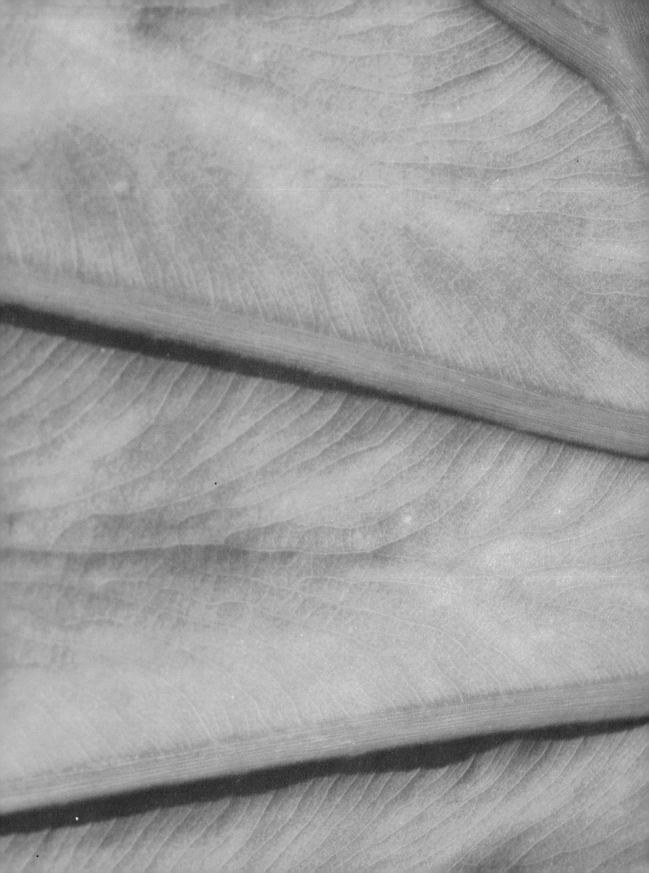

Mariel's Kitchen

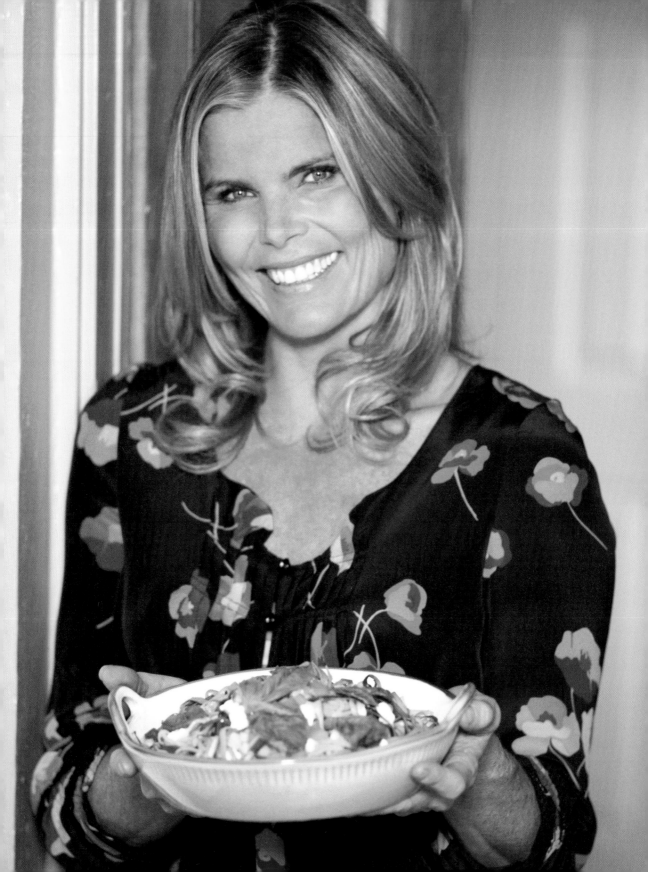

Introduction

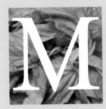**M**y kitchen is the heart of my home. It is where my day begins and where my day ends. It's where I can feel the pulse of my world. Every person, and every animal, in my family passes through the kitchen at some point, and they show what they need without any pretense. There's something about the primal activity that happens in the kitchen—that very necessary feeding of body and brain—that makes people, and small dogs, very honest.

First thing, last thing, and throughout the day when I'm home, my kitchen is also where I check in with myself. Food is the centering point; it's the foundation from which everything else—productivity, creativity, loving, and evolving—can start.

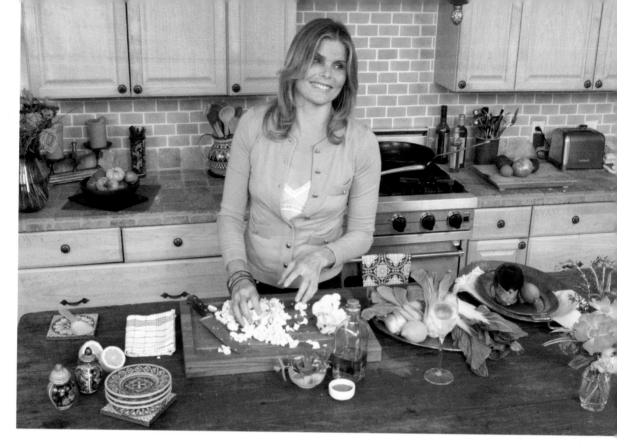

Not long ago, I had the experience of befriending a new kitchen. Medium-sized, unpretentious, and instantly welcoming, my kitchen quickly became the heart of my new home. The floor is lined in fat clay tiles that stay cool under bare feet. The counter space is modest, so I keep it clutter free. I furnished it simply with a big farmhouse table and one cozy armchair; daughters and friends have somewhere to sit while I tear pale lettuce leaves or mix dough with my hands. It's the opposite of a perfect, designer kitchen; those rooms leave me cold. There's little appeal in marble surfaces never splashed with yellow olive oil, or state-of-the-art sinks never graced by blackened pans. A kitchen only comes alive when it's used.

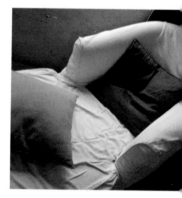

An armchair in the kitchen is an invitation to sit and talk.

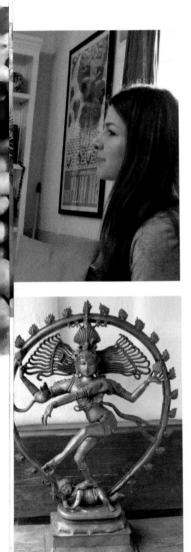

The feeling in my kitchen is a reflection of my food: easy and comfortable; integrated into a busy life. I appreciate the gourmet chefs of the world, but part of what makes food satisfying for me is simplicity. A piece of fish with a fresh veggie salsa requires just minutes of dicing. Fresh herbs, mixed in unusual combinations like cumin and mint, are enough to excite my senses. Shaking a bottle of my own freshly made dressing, as rich as store bought but infinitely more lively, never fails to give me a smile.

This simplicity around food is also designed by necessity. Of all the things I do to stay happy and balanced, healthy eating gets top priority. To happen three times a day, it's got to be streamlined. This news surprises some, who know my passion for yoga, exercise, and spiritual practice. Surely, they think, those things are more sacred than what I have for lunch? But none of them can happen without the energy and clarity that comes from eating well. And as I've found over and over, food is the first teacher of all the qualities these other practices develop—awareness, acceptance, gratitude, and grace. Wake up to what you put in your body, notice how your food or drink feels, how it heals or hurts, and you will inevitably wake up to your whole life.

It took a few decades to come to this understanding, but now my definition of healthy eating comes more from common-sense wisdom than the encyclopedic knowledge of nutrition stored in my mind. When we prepare food fresh and eat it slowly, we know when we are full and we get more nourishment from it. Physically and emotionally, in our cells and our spirits, we're happier and more sustainable life is often through the kitchen door. Whole foods cooked from their natural, raw state are better for our bodies and the planet than packaged meals and snacks. Farmers' Markets let us increase our nutritional intake with local, pesticide-free foods, and as a side effect, decrease our carbon footprint. Spending more on meat, dairy, and fish from better sources and eating it far less often, as humans historically have done, is more sustainable all around. As you'll discover in this book, I am a passionate advocate for making deliberate choices about animal protein. Start by asking your supermarket where their products came from, and then vote for change with your dollar, picking organic, grass-fed meats; humane-certified, hormone-free poultry; and wild-caught or healthily farmed fish when you can. (See the Resources section at the end of this book for help.) Quality, not quantity, is my credo for these foods—and you won't go hungry when vibrant vegetables and nurturing side dishes make up the rest of the plate. At this time in our evolution, we don't have a choice but to live more consciously; the planet and the economy are asking us to do more with fewer resources, to return to a simpler way of being. Let your breakfast, lunch, or dinner show you the way.

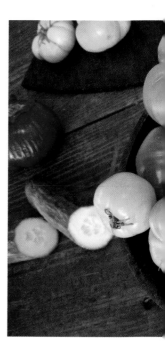

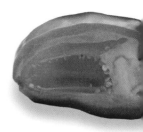

Eating simply and seasonally is, thankfully, delicious. It satisfies that instinctual craving for thick, hot soup on a winter night, or a bowl of crisp, just-picked vegetables in spring. It draws our attention to smells and textures we sometimes miss when things get more complex. Furthermore, it lets us enjoy the rituals around food rather than getting flustered by the preparation. Use what looks freshest at the market; make creative substitutions if need be.

Buy with your eyes; pick out the produce that looks most vibrant.

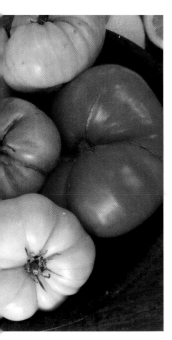

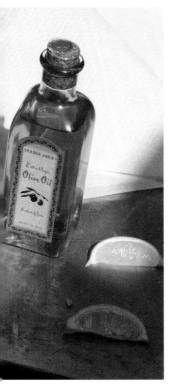

Touch and handle the produce, considering how to use it. All this I find incredibly calming. Whether we cook and eat alone or surrounded by others, when we keep it simple, we can gracefully find a way to turn the act of eating into a precious and nurturing ritual; something that enhances our hidden, yet already peaceful, sense of well-being.

The first section of this book features my fifteen core recipes, those everyday standards that ensure my kitchen runs with the least effort and stays largely free of packaged or processed store-bought foods. That's followed by a selection of my favorite meals and snacks for each time of year. There's no need to be constrained by this seasonal format. Pick and choose dishes to try from the whole book according to what appeals to you and which ingredients you'll be easily able to find. Mix and match the protein dishes with vegetable sides or salads for a larger meal. Sometimes you'll use frozen vegetables, fruits, and produce, meaning many recipes work year-round. But let the seasons inspire you to cook with what's freshest, and tune in to what your body wants to eat that day. Approaching food from a quiet place lets your intuition guide your choices; you may be surprised by how it naturally points you to the local and seasonal, those things bursting with ripeness and flavor.

This book is also a gentle invitation to experience some other dietary practices that have been central to my own health path: fewer starchy vegetables, no wheat, and minimal grains in general, because of these foods' inflammatory effect on tissue and joints and their destabilizing effect on blood sugar. You can work around this by adding your favorite sides—though try substituting quinoa or brown rice for pasta, potatoes, and bread if you feel inspired. And where I use rice flour, you can still go ahead with wheat.

The use of dairy is light throughout because I find it heavy on the body. Organic goat or sheep dairy products are always an option, as they're easier to digest. (I've found myself cutting down on milk products for ethical reasons too; the ramifications of industrialized dairy farming, even organic, don't sit well with me.) And though the desserts featured are free of refined sugars, they are still treats, not meals in themselves. Enjoy them in small portions and savor every bite! Eating this way may require you to change some habits and expectations of what a meal should be, but your palate and your energy levels will register a difference.

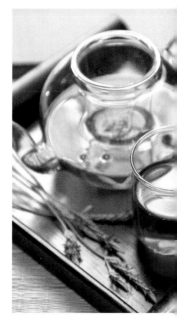

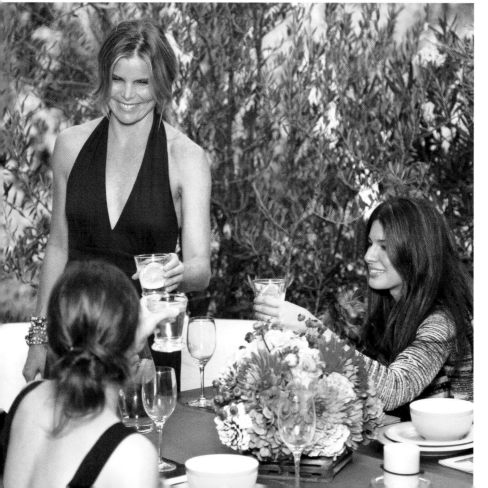

Small rituals like making your favorite tea or having friends around the table begin to change your relationship to food. You slow down and get the most satisfaction from it.

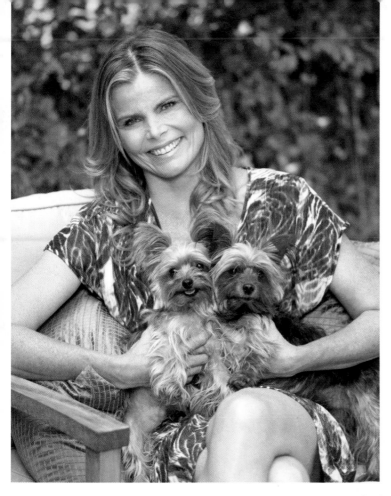

Try making a few of these meals each week. Before you know it, there'll be a repertoire of easy meals at your fingertips. Some of them will probably become the signatures of your own kitchen. Most importantly, let them inspire you to create joyously through cooking! We know that eating food is a necessity, not a choice. It's a basic need, and in our busy lives it can easily become stripped of feeling. But the kind of food we eat and the way we prepare it *is* our choice, every day. That's why my kitchen feels the way it does: grounded and calm, a place to be grateful. I choose to fill it with simple, whole foods, rich in color and flavor; I choose to cook them easily but mindfully. With each simple meal I say thank you to the great source it comes from—the earth beneath my feet—and it returns the favor, sustaining not just my body, but also my spirit.

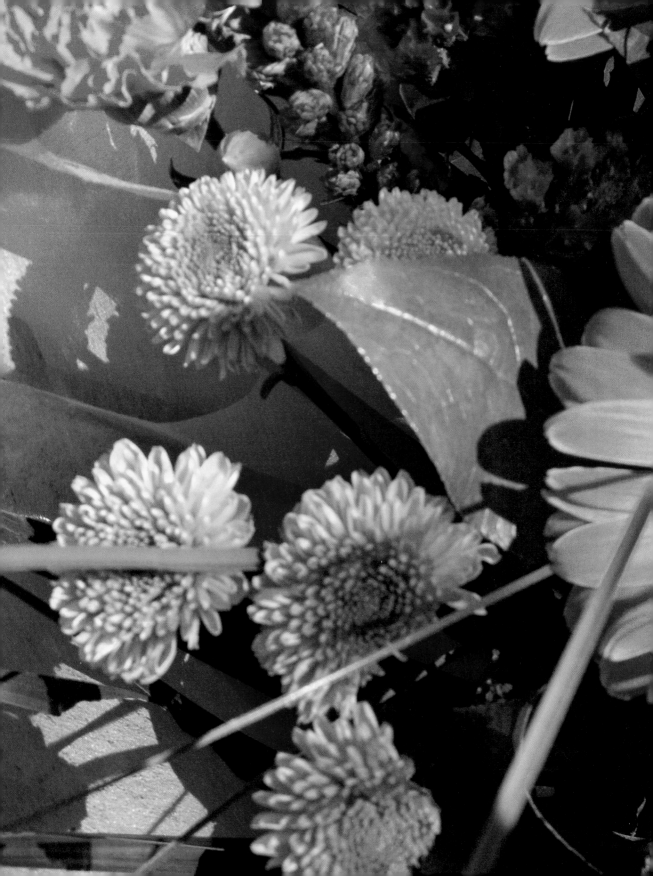

Essentials

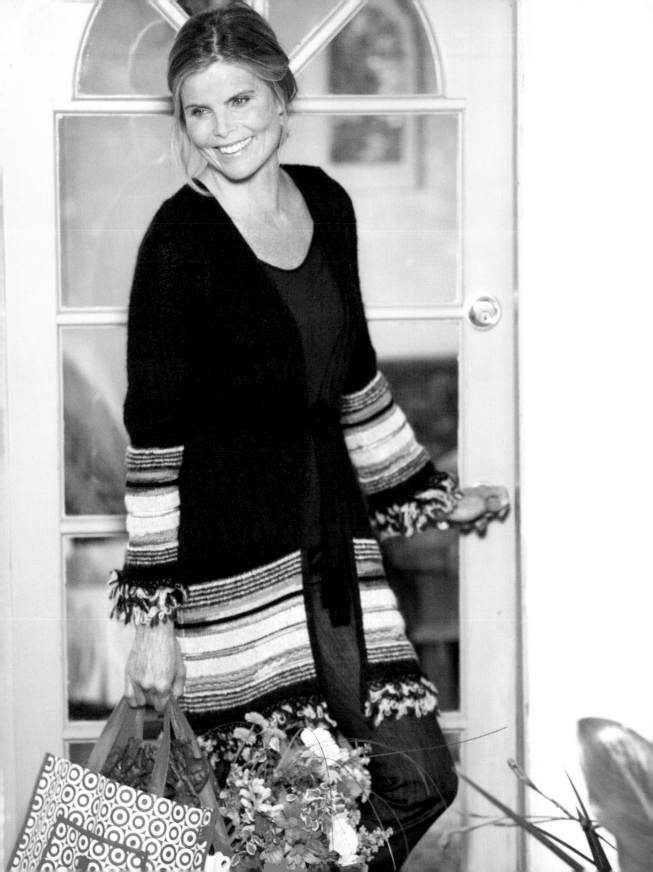

Pantry Essentials

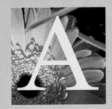A simple, seasonal kitchen doesn't demand cupboards groaning with exotic ingredients. When the emphasis is on fresh foods whenever possible, the support team of staple goods is important, but it can be a relatively lean collection. You don't need to invest in an entire new pantry to start cooking the meals in this book. A few strategic purchases will get you going. Watch what happens. Slowly your pantry will get a makeover and things that once seemed a little odd will become part of everyday routine.

Some of these ingredients you may not have used before; others are fairly standard but are better found outside the regular supermarket aisle, where they can be overpriced, overprocessed, or nutritionally lacking. Often these items found their way into my pantry initially for health reasons and then got invited back because they work brilliantly and taste great. Now they're old friends.

Coconut oil

The oil I cook with most, coconut oil doesn't oxidize at high heat, which causes cell damage (remember, we want *anti*oxidants in our diet), like other vegetable oils. Its fat is burned off fast, and it has powerful antimicrobial properties. It adds a light, but not overpowering, flavor. Look for organic and unrefined brands like Nutiva. Spectrum is also widely available.

Whey protein isolate

A derivative of dairy, whey protein isolate powder packs protein into smoothies. I also use it for frozen desserts. Beware of brands that have high sugar content (they will say fructose, sucrose, maltodextrin), or worse—chemicals like aspartame. The Jay Robb brand, which is sweetened only with stevia and is widely available in healthy supermarkets, works best. The vanilla powder is my staple, but the unflavored version is used in some recipes here.

Xylosweet

The Xylosweet brand of xylitol—a natural, nonsugar sweetener made from birch trees and other natural sources—is adaptable to all kinds of dishes and won't elevate blood sugar. It's better than stevia for

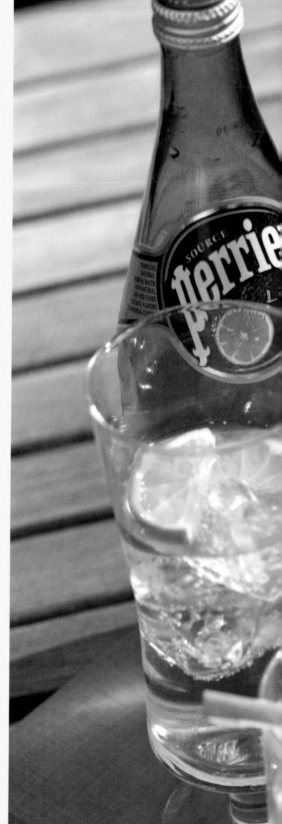

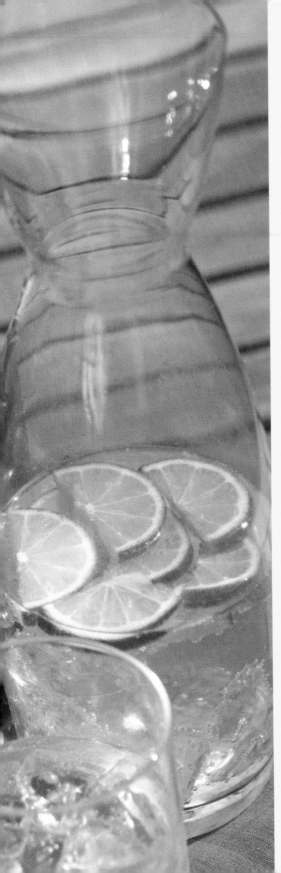

cooking and baking, since stevia can lend baked goods a bitter taste, and is available in large bags. Some people have digestive discomfort if they eat too much—be aware of your body's response. It's also handy to have SweetLeaf stevia for drinks and smoothies. It's another natural, nonsugar sweetener, made from a South American plant.

Brown rice flour, coconut flour, almond meal

These three wheat substitutes are used as thickeners in some recipes and in place of wheat in baking. Almond meal, also called almond flour, gives a delicious coating to chicken or fish before baking. Coconut flour has a slight nutty flavor and, like the others, is nicely low-carb and high in fiber. Bob's Red Mill and Authentic Foods are the brands I usually buy.

Other oils

In addition to regular virgin olive oil for cooking, it's nice to have premium oils to use with discernment—like great chocolate, small amounts go a long way. The deeper-colored oils drizzle beautifully on steamed or grilled vegetables, salads, and fish in small amounts (they're too precious for frying). A bottle of walnut oil, a top-of-the-line olive oil, and macadamia oil, kept out of the light, will start your collection. In addition, Omega-3-rich flax oil—for smoothies—is kept in the fridge.

Vinegars

Alongside apple cider and white balsamic, ume plum vinegar is a tangy, salty variety that comes from the Japanese process of pickling plums. It's great sprinkled on cooked or raw vegetables, in salad dressing, or as a dip.

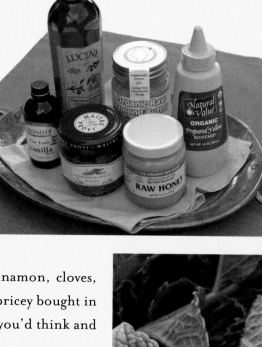

Herbs and spices

Until you have a full collection of dried herbs, a jar of herbs de Provençe serves many needs. Separate jars of thyme, tarragon, paprika, cayenne, and rosemary are a must, as are cumin, turmeric, curry powder, cinnamon, cloves, and ginger. Fresh herbs are always ideal, but can be pricey bought in small packets. Growing them indoors is easier than you'd think and saves a lot of money.

Vanilla and almond extracts

You'll need vanilla and almond extracts for the Blisscuit recipe, which is the foundation of several other recipes in the book. Pick up shredded coconut also—if you have a bulk section at your health-food store, it's an affordable way to get it—and xanthan gum, a natural thickener.

Raw cashews, walnuts, almonds, Brazil nuts

Best bought in bulk, raw nuts are great for snacking, making nut butter, and are easy to roast yourself at low heat with no oil on them. Some prefer to soak their nuts overnight to make them more digestible. Don't do this if you're planning to make the Sweet Roasted or Spicy Mixed Nut snacks.

A few strategic purchases will soon become a healthy new pantry.

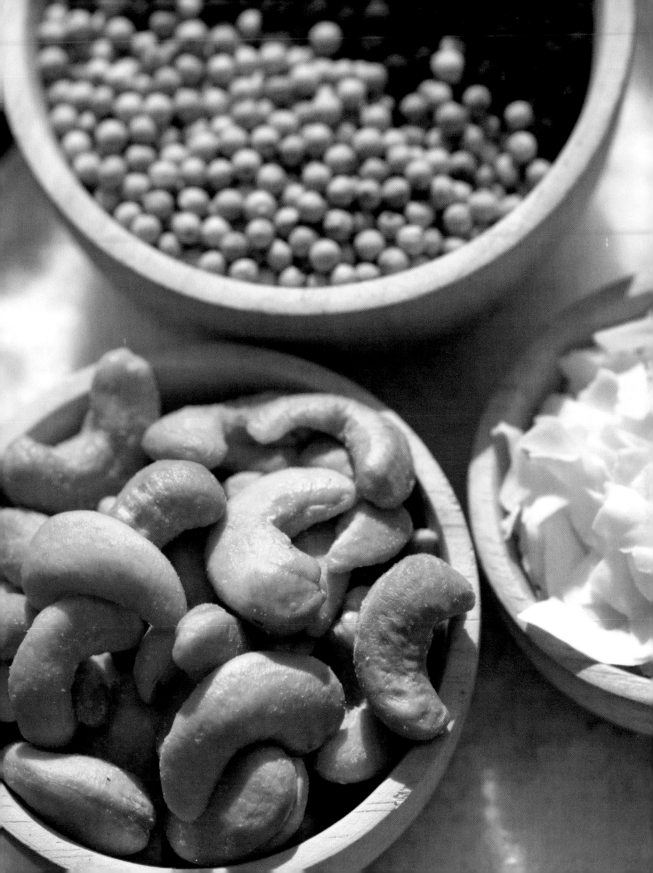

Salt

Regular table salt is highly refined and lacks essential nutrients. Good, coarse sea salt is a better bet for cooking and for your health. But above all, I like pink Himalayan salt because it is completely unrefined and much more pure, leaving all the key minerals you need intact.

Quinoa

Nutty and light, quinoa is a cinch to cook, taking fifteen minutes in contrast to brown rice's forty-five. It's full of the essential proteins and amino acids we need to function, but not as sugary as refined white starches, so it's great as a side or as the basis for a satisfying salad. Rinse it well before cooking. I even use it in a hot breakfast cereal called Quinoa Mush on cold mornings.

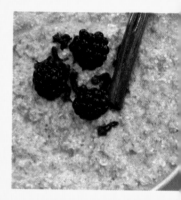

Teas

A whole shelf of my pantry is devoted to teas. Where other people have wine collections, I like my leaves. Having noticed how caffeine affects me for the worse, I prefer rooibos, decaffeinated green teas, and unusual finds like Japanese buckwheat tea. And I always buy loose leaves, not tea bags. Making a pot of tea is the most immediate way to slow down and bring a little ritual into life. The leaves also work well iced in hot weather.

Mustard

Keep several types of mustard in your pantry, including a natural yellow mustard and a grainy dijon, delicious on all kinds of protein and the basis for easy salad dressings.

Coconut milk

I always have a few cans of this to whip up the Coconut Whey Frozen Dessert and to speedily make my Cashew Sauce with curry powder to pour over steamed vegetables and rice.

Organic/non-genetically modified soy and almond milks

Stocking up on organic soy and almond milks makes it simple to blend up a smoothie when you're hungry, instead of reaching for a boxed or processed snack.

Frozen berries

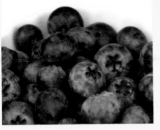

These live in the freezer but are still a pantry essential, used in many recipes. Prices at some national chain markets can be good, so look around. (If you're lucky to live in an area with abundant summertime berries growing wild, do a big day of picking and freeze them for the year.)

See Resources for my favorite brands and sources.

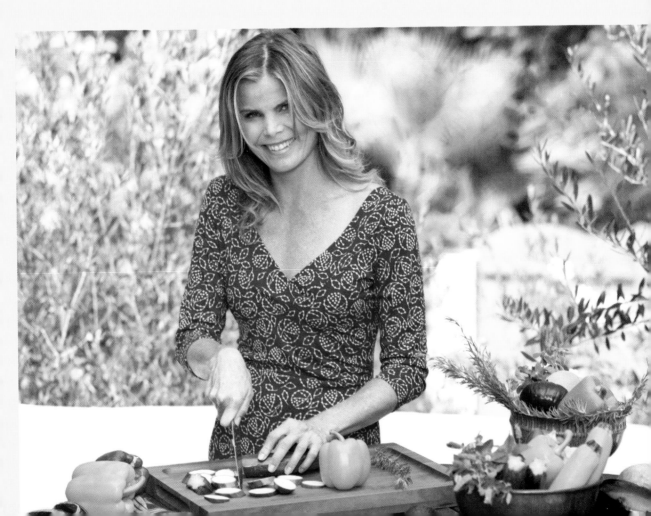

Seasoning Chart

FOOD	SEASONING
Beans, dry	Bay leaf, black pepper, cumin, garlic, parsley, thyme
Beans, green	Basil, black pepper, garlic, marjoram, savory, thyme
Beef	Bay leaf, black pepper, chili powder, cumin, garlic, ginger, thyme
Beets	Basil, dill, ginger, mint, mustard, parsley
Carrots	Cinnamon, cloves, dill, mint, nutmeg, parsley, savory, tarragon, thyme
Cauliflower	Chives, curry powder, nutmeg, parsley
Chicken	Basil, bay leaf, chives, cilantro, cinnamon, cloves, cumin, curry powder, garlic, ginger, marjoram, mustard, rosemary, sage, tarragon, thyme
Corn	Basil, chives, chili powder, dill, mint, parsley
Duck	Parsley, sage, thyme
Eggplant	Basil, cilantro, cumin, garlic, parsley, thyme
Fish	Basil, bay leaf, chervil, chives, cilantro, cumin, curry, dill, marjoram, mint, mustard, oregano, paprika, parsley, saffron, savory, tarragon, thyme
Lamb	Cumin, curry, garlic, mint, oregano, rosemary
Peas	Basil, marjoram, mint, parsley, savory, tarragon
Pork	Allspice, bay leaf, cumin, fennel, garlic, ginger, marjoram, mustard, rosemary, sage, thyme
Potatoes	Chives, dill, garlic, rosemary, parsley, thyme
Spinach	Curry, garlic, nutmeg
Squash, summer	Basil, chives, garlic, marjoram, oregano, parsley, savory
Squash, winter	Allspice, cinnamon, cloves, mace, nutmeg
Tomatoes	Basil, chives, garlic, marjoram, oregano, parsley, savory, tarragon, thyme
Turkey	Bay leaf, rosemary, sage, savory
Veal	Basil, bay leaf, lemon, parsley, savory, tarragon, thyme

Produce Available All Year

Apples	Garlic
Avocados	Green onions
Bananas	Jicama
Beets	Kale
Bell peppers	Lemons
Bok choy	Leeks
Broccoli	Lettuce
Butternut squash	Limes
Cabbage	Mushrooms
Carrots	Onions
Cauliflower	Pineapple
Celery	Radishes
Chiles	Spinach
Cucumbers	Tomatillos
Eggplant	Tomatoes
Fennel	Zucchini

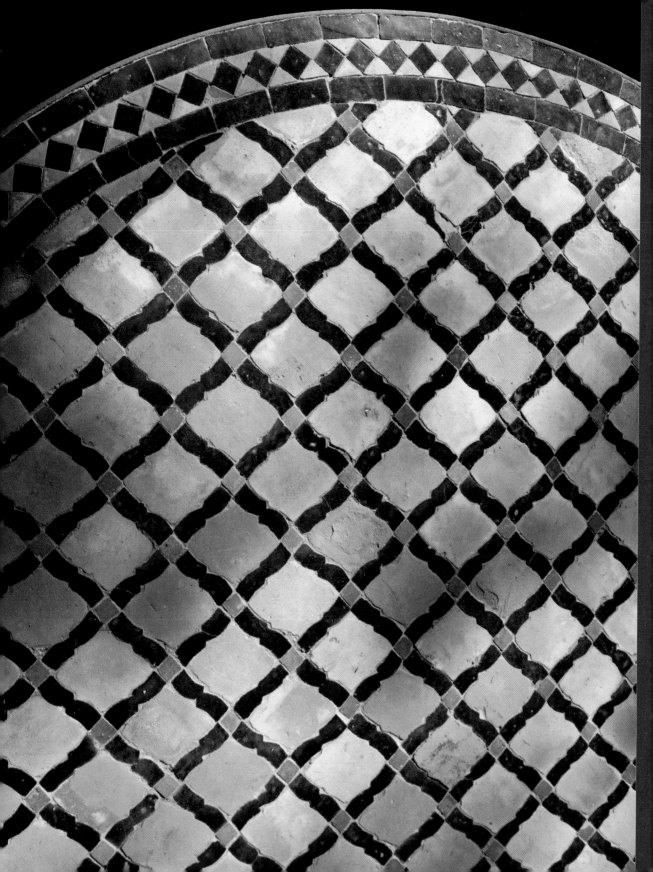

Mariel's Core Recipes

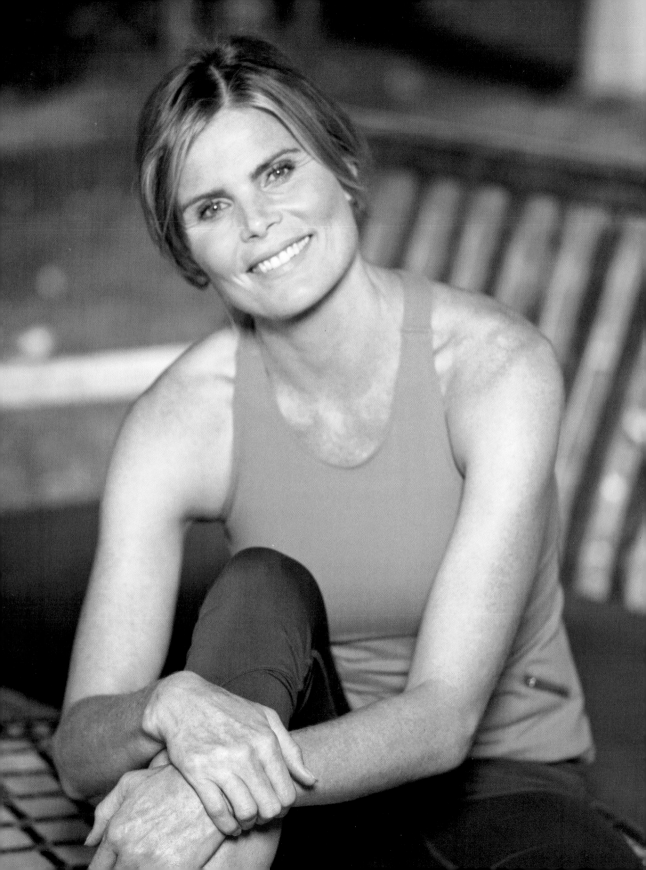

Breakfast Smoothie

SERVES 2

- 1 cup fresh organic orange juice
- 1 cup fresh organic carrot juice
- 2 cups organic GMO-free soy milk or almond milk
- 2 small organic bananas, peeled and quartered
- 2 scoops whey protein isolate powder (about 4 tablespoons)
- 2 teaspoons Xylosweet, optional

1. Combine all ingredients with about 2 cups ice cubes in a blender. Blend until combined and frothy. Serve immediately.

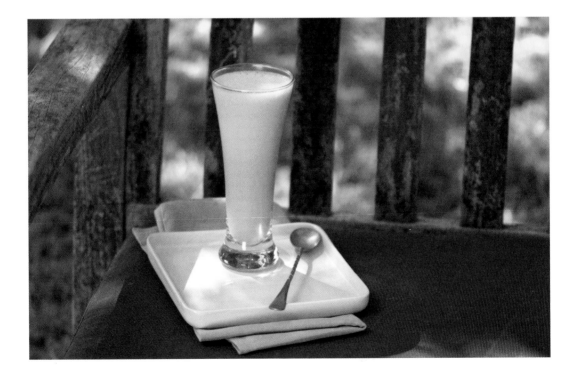

Breakfast Pudding

1   (10-ounce) bag frozen blueberries

1   organic avocado

1   teaspoon flax oil

2   scoops vanilla whey protein isolate powder

2   limes, juiced

¼–½   cup boiling water, more or less as needed

1. Combine all ingredients in a blender and blend until smooth. Add boiling water as necessary to reach desired consistency.

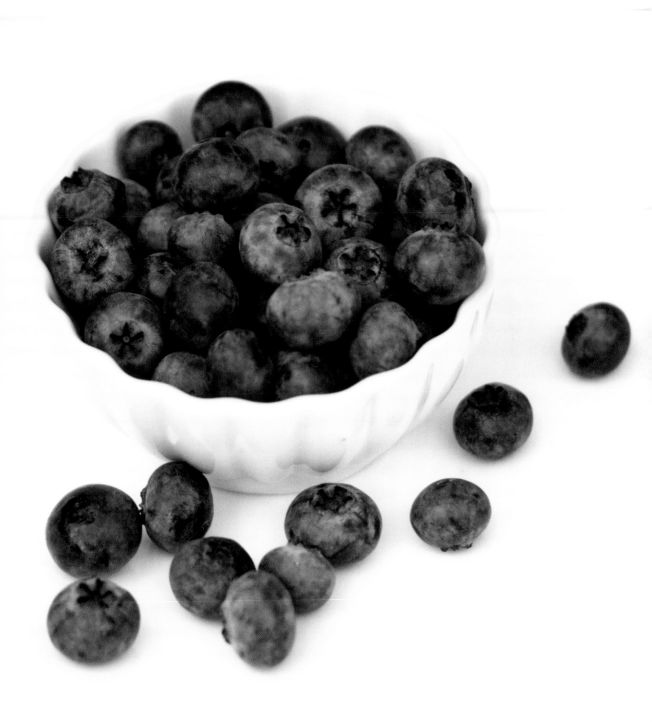

Spinach Pancakes

These beautiful green pancakes can be used as tortilla-like wraps or rolled with fillings for savory crepes. These are also used in place of pasta to make my Spinach and Mushroom Lasagna (pg. 230).

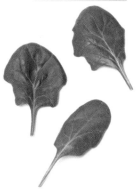

4 large eggs

1 (10-ounce) package frozen, organic spinach, thawed and drained

2 cloves garlic, chopped

⅔ cup low-fat milk or almond milk

1 tablespoon olive oil

2 tablespoons almond meal flour

½ teaspoon sea salt

Cooking spray

1. Combine eggs, spinach, garlic, milk, oil, flour, and salt in a blender or food processor and blend until well combined.

2. Coat a 6- to 8-inch nonstick pan with nonstick cooking spray and heat over medium heat. Pour a small amount of batter in the pan and spread to coat bottom. Cook pancake until the batter bubbles evenly and the bottom is browned, and then flip to cook the other side until browned. Remove to a platter and repeat until all batter is used. Serve immediately or freeze individually for later use.

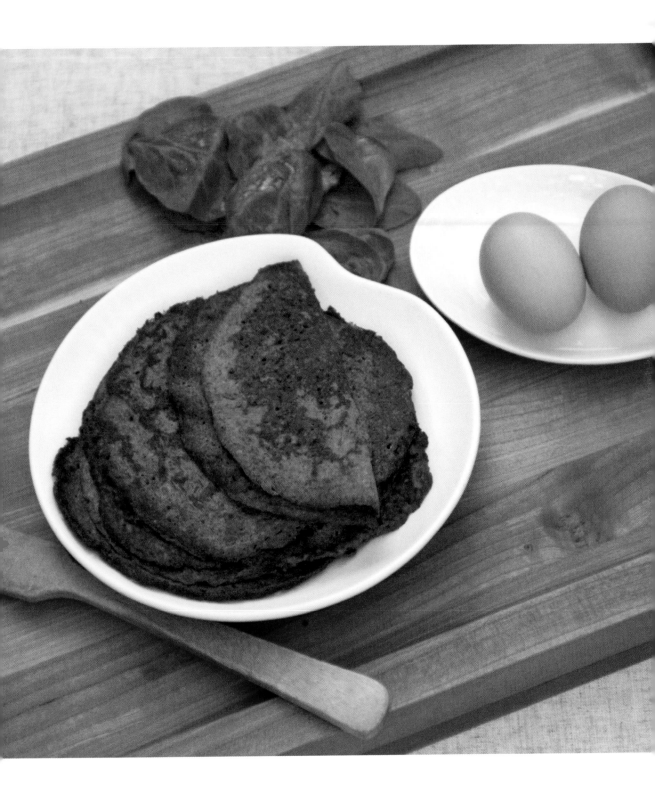

Everyday Mustard Dressing

This easy
dressing can
be tossed with
salads, used as
a sauce for fish
or chicken, or
even used as a
dip for veggies.
For a flavorful
variation, throw
in a tablespoon
of fresh basil,
tarragon, or dill.

Keep on hand
for salads,
sandwiches, or
dipping sauce
for snacks.

MAKES ABOUT ½ CUP

2 tablespoons Dijon mustard

2 teaspoons freshly squeezed lemon juice

1 tablespoon white balsamic vinegar

¼ cup olive oil

1. Place all ingredients in a blender or food processor
   and process until creamy.

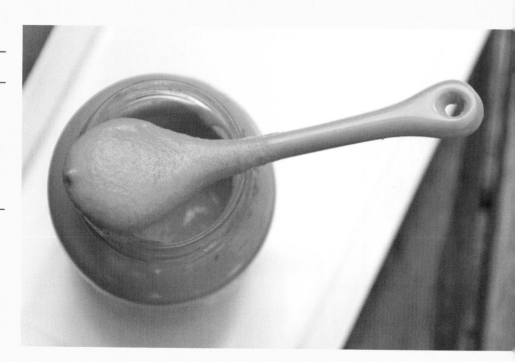

Spicy Mixed Nuts

- 1 cup whole raw nuts
- 2 teaspoons coconut oil
- ¼ teaspoon curry powder
- ¼ teaspoon dried thyme
- ⅛ teaspoon ground cumin
- ⅛ teaspoon salt
- ⅛ teaspoon cayenne pepper
- ⅛ teaspoon paprika

1. Preheat oven to 300°F.
2. Toss nuts and coconut oil together to coat.
3. Place curry powder, thyme, cumin, salt, pepper, and paprika in a medium bowl and stir to combine. Add nuts and toss to coat evenly in spice mixture.
4. Spread on a baking sheet and bake until nuts just begin to brown, about 20 minutes.
5. Serve while still warm or at room temperature.

Use a mixture of your favorite nuts in this spicy recipe. Walnuts, almonds, pecans, and hazelnuts all work great. These will keep for up to 3 days if stored in an airtight container at room temperature.

For an herbed nut variation, replace the curry, cumin, cayenne, and paprika with an additional ¼ teaspoon dried thyme, ¼ teaspoon dried rosemary, ¼ teaspoon lemon pepper, and ⅛ teaspoon ground sage.

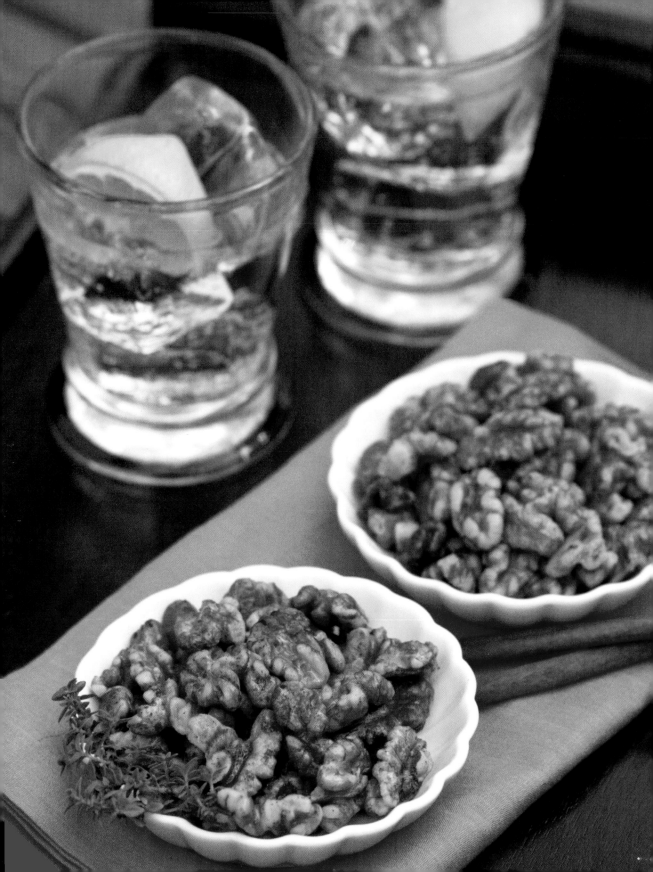

Sweet Roasted Nuts

MAKES 1 CUP

  1 cup whole raw nuts

  2 teaspoons coconut oil

  ¾ teaspoon ground cinnamon

  ⅛ teaspoon ground clove

     Pinch of ground ginger

  1 teaspoon Xylosweet

1. Preheat oven to 300°F.

2. Toss nuts and coconut oil together to coat.

3. Place cinnamon, clove, ginger, and Xylosweet in a medium bowl and stir to combine. Add nuts and toss to coat evenly.

4. Spread on a baking sheet and bake until nuts just begin to brown, about 20 minutes.

5. Serve while still warm or at room temperature.

These sweet nuts make a great snack. Or coarsely chop and sprinkle on yogurt, cereal, or ice cream. You can even add these to salads.

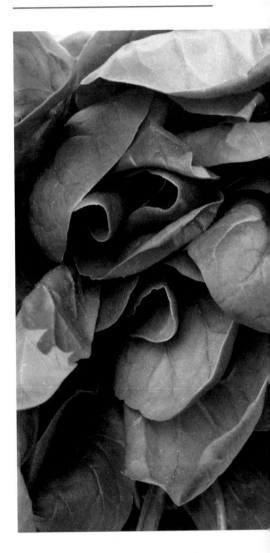

Basic Blisscuits

This makes enough dough for about 60 Blisscuits—make the whole recipe and freeze the leftovers.

2 cups almond meal

1 cup plus 2 tablespoons whey protein isolate powder

1 cup plus 1 tablespoon Xylosweet

½ cup finely shredded coconut

3 tablespoons coconut flour

3 tablespoons brown rice flour

2 ½ tablespoons ground cinnamon

1 ¾ teaspoons baking powder

2 ¼ teaspoons xanthan gum

1 cup coconut oil

3 large egg whites

1 ¼ teaspoons vanilla extract

¾ teaspoon almond extract

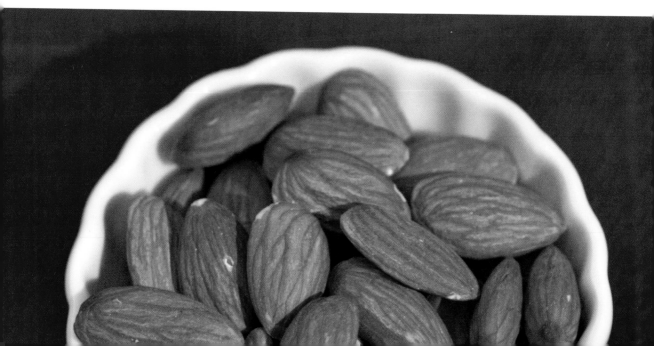

1. Preheat oven to 300°F. Cover two large baking sheets with parchment paper and set aside.

2. Place all dry ingredients in a large bowl and mix together well. In a medium bowl whisk together coconut oil, egg whites, and vanilla and almond extracts. Pour wet ingredients into dry and mix together well.

3. Roll out dough to ¼ inch thick and cut into 2-inch squares. Or form into 2-inch patties, ¼ inch thick, with your hands. Place on prepared baking sheets and bake until golden, 15 to 20 minutes.

4. Let cool before storing in an airtight container for up to 4 days or freeze for up to a month.

Divide dough into 1-cup amounts and wrap tightly in plastic wrap, then in foil. Blisscuit dough can be frozen for up to 2 months. This way you can defrost a cup at a time and bake fresh Blisscuits whenever you like.

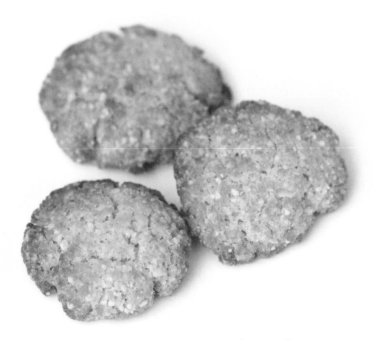

Blisscuit variations

for 8 ounces (1 cup) of basic Blisscuit dough:

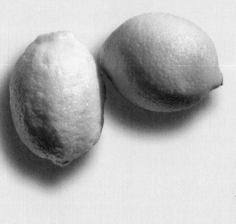

Lemon Poppy Seed Blisscuit

Add

1	tablespoon freshly squeezed lemon juice
2	teaspoons finely grated lemon zest
2	teaspoons poppy seeds

Chocolate Blisscuit

Add

3	tablespoons unsweetened cocoa powder
1	tablespoon coconut oil
⅛	teaspoon sea salt

Adding a small amount of cream cheese, mascarpone, ricotta or neufatchel cheese (1–2 tablespoons per cup of dough) will strengthen it enough to make a crust or crackers.

Savory Cheese Blisscuit

Add

2	tablespoons organic goat cheese
¼	teaspoon sea salt
¼	teaspoon freshly ground black pepper

3. Shape the turkey sausage mixture into 28 patties about 1 ½ inches in diameter. Heat the 2 tablespoons oil in a large skillet and brown the patties over medium heat on both sides, about 2 minutes per side. Reduce the heat to medium low, cover the skillet and cook, turning the patties occasionally, until they are cooked through, about 4 minutes. (You may have to do this in a few batches.)

4. Serve immediately or freeze in individual containers to reheat for a quick snack.

Eat these for breakfast, lunch, or dinner. The small, bite-size nuggets make for pre-portioned protein when you need it.

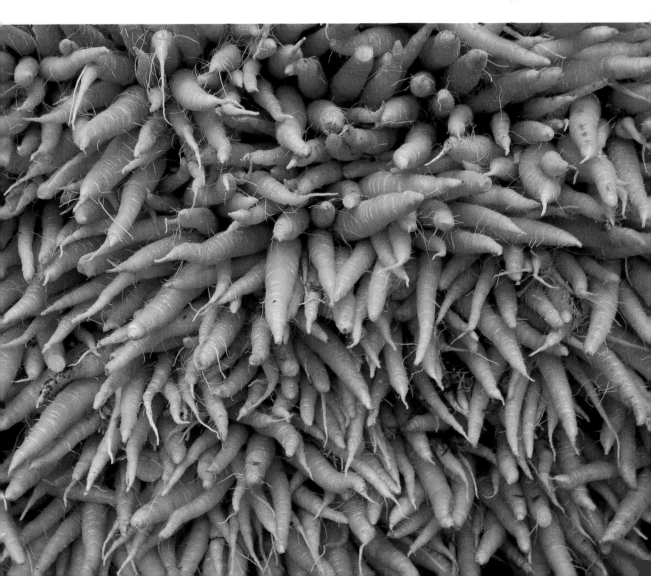

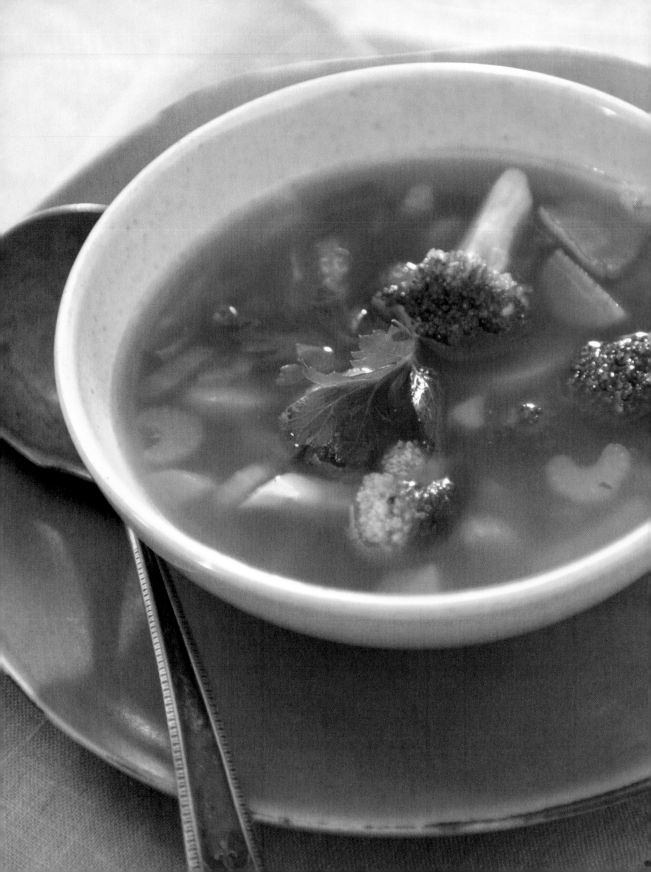

All-Season Vegetable Soup

SERVES 4–6

1 tablespoon olive oil

½ small yellow onion, diced

1 medium organic carrot, cut in half length-wise and sliced

1 medium organic celery stalk, sliced

2 garlic cloves, minced

6 cups quality organic vegetable broth

3 cups chopped, mixed, organic seasonal vegetables of your choice

1 cup broccoli florets

1 ½ tablespoons finely chopped fresh basil

1 tablespoon finely chopped fresh parsley

½ teaspoon finely chopped fresh thyme

¼ teaspoon dried red pepper flakes

Sea salt

Freshly ground black pepper

1. Heat oil in a large, heavy pot or Dutch oven over medium heat.

   Add onion, carrot, and celery and sauté until softened.

   Add garlic and sauté just until fragrant.

2. Add broth and vegetables and bring to a boil. Reduce heat.
   Simmer until vegetables are barely tender.

3. Add herbs and season with salt and pepper. Serve immediately.
   Refrigerate leftovers for up to 2 days.

Coconut Whey Frozen Dessert

SERVES 6–8

This recipe can be easily altered by adding chunky or pureed fruit, carob chips or powder, toasted coconut, unsweetened apple butter, fig spread, nut butters or chopped nuts, or any type of liquid or powdered extract or flavoring.

3 cups coconut water or coconut milk

4 ½ scoops whey protein isolate powder (1 ⅔ cups)

1. Mix coconut water and whey powder together well. Place in an ice cream maker and freeze according to manufacturer's directions.

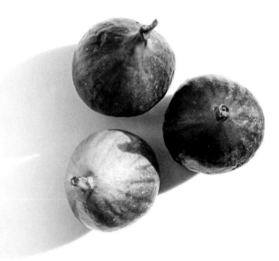

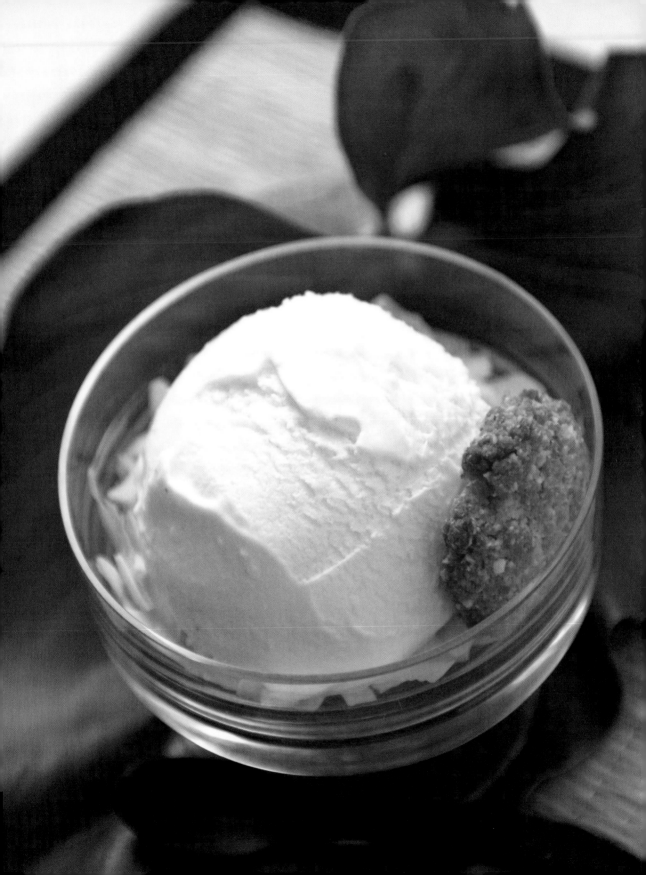

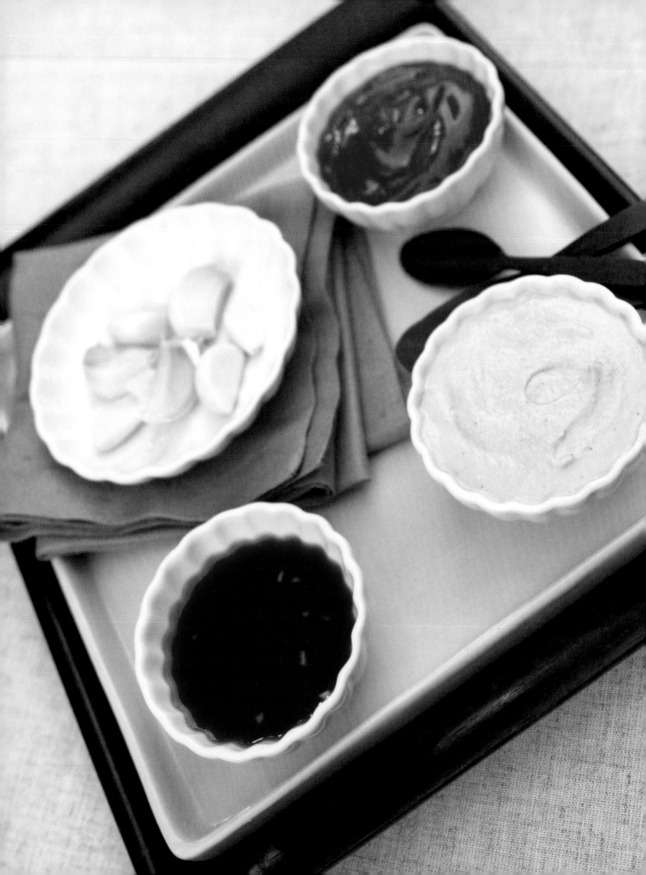

Sugar-Free Ketchup

MAKES 6 CUPS

- 2 cups apple cider vinegar
- 1 (28-ounce) can organic tomato sauce
- 1 (12-ounce) can organic tomato paste
- 4 tablespoons Xylosweet
- 1 cinnamon stick
- 1 teaspoon freshly ground black pepper
- 1 teaspoon freshly ground all-spice
- ½ teaspoon Worcestershire sauce
- 1 teaspoon fresh lemon juice
  Salt

1. Combine vinegar, tomato sauce, tomato paste, Xylosweet, cinnamon stick, pepper, all-spice, Worcestershire sauce, and lemon juice in a medium saucepan over high heat. Bring to a boil, reduce heat, and simmer for about 20 minutes.
2. Remove from heat, extract cinnamon stick, and add salt to taste.
3. Keep chilled in an airtight container until ready to use.

All-Purpose Marinade

MAKES ¾ CUP

- ¼ cup soy sauce
- ¼ cup freshly squeezed orange juice
- 2 tablespoons freshly squeezed lime juice
- 2 tablespoons coconut oil
- 1 clove garlic
- ⅛ teaspoon Xylosweet, more or less to taste

1. Place all ingredients in a blender or food processor and process until creamy.

This recipe uses fresh orange and lime juice. Zest the skin of the orange and lime to add more flavor to this marinade.

Creamy Avocado Lime Dressing

MAKES ABOUT ⅓ CUP

This dressing is just the right combination of creamy and tangy for seafood salads. It's also great on any cooked seafood.

1   avocado, peeled and pitted

1 ½   tablespoons freshly squeezed lime juice

Sea salt

Freshly ground black pepper

I. Place avocado and lime juice in a small food processor and blend until smooth. Add a little cold water to thin if desired. Season with salt and pepper.

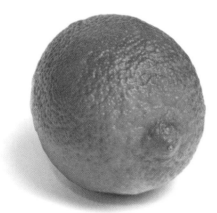

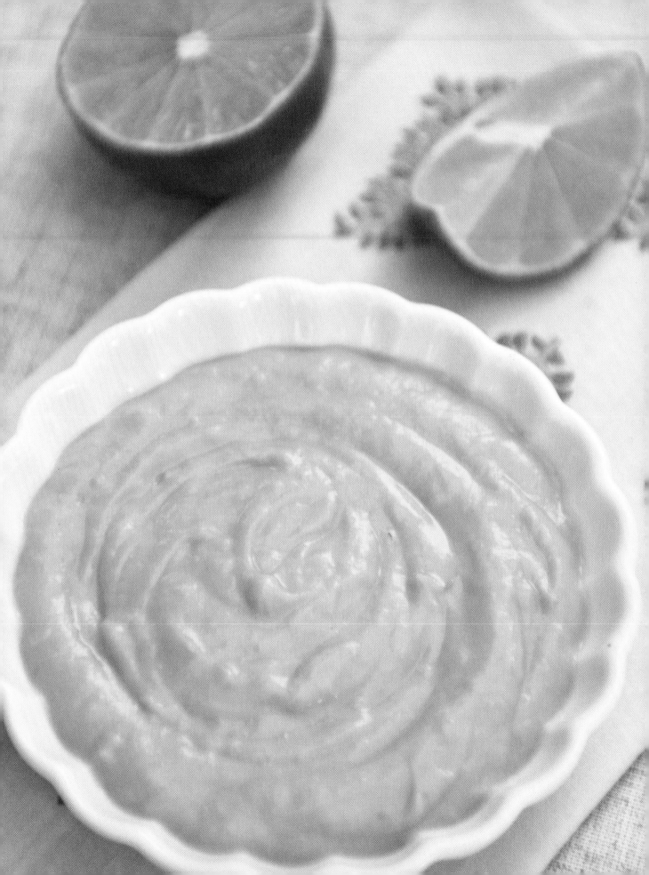

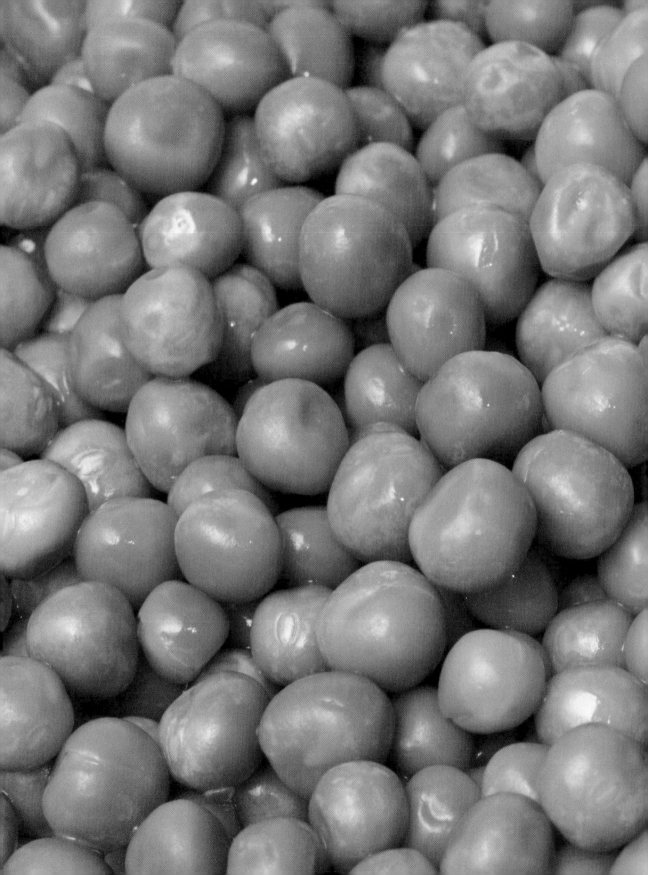

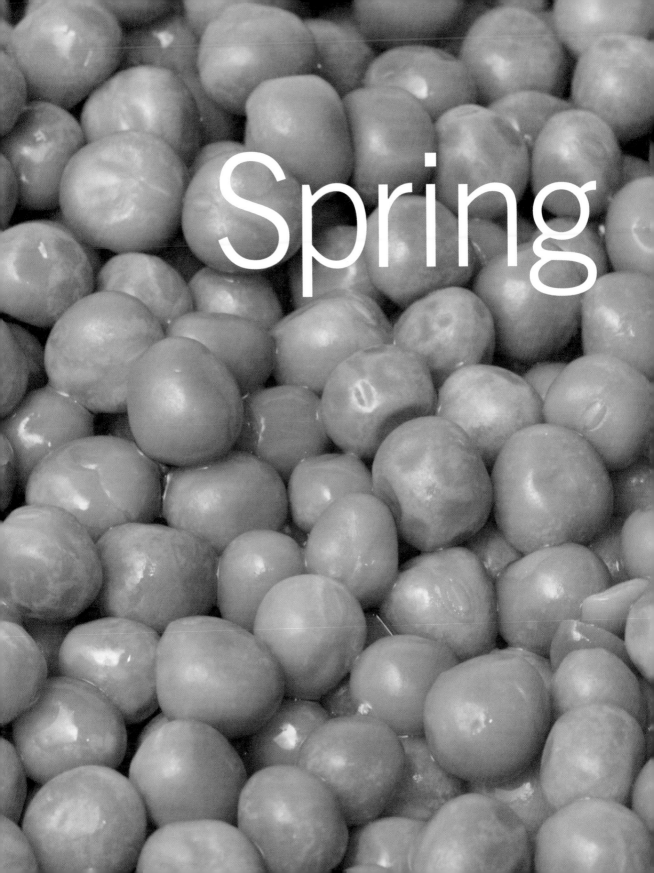

Spring

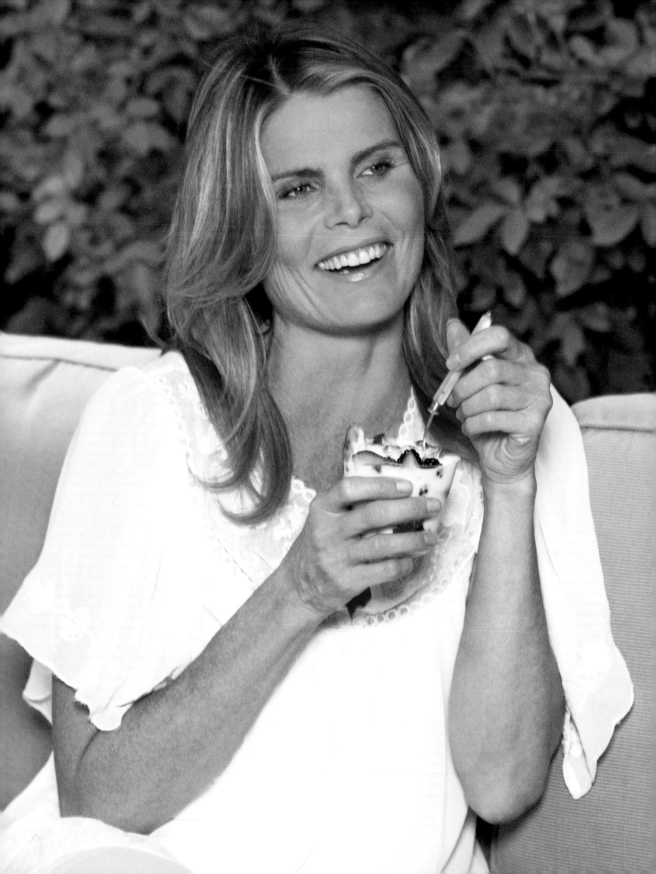

Fresh Colors, Delicate Tastes

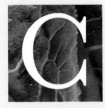ome springtime, I want to feel new. The heaviest sweaters are put away and after a few months of wintery stews and soups, it's time to lighten up in the kitchen as well. Raw foods appear on my plate; as new shoots burst through the earth, bodies crave that same energy. The senses are ready for invigoration, not just cold-weather nurturing! A tangle of watercress scattered on a shrimp wrap tickles the tongue with its tiny curls of new plant life. The watery feel of cucumbers and jicama—a turnip-like vegetable with a texture like pear—is refreshing as spring rain.

But the best thing about spring eating is the rainbow of colors that burst from the soil and the sea. A long winter can get us stuck in a rut; colorful food shakes us out of it. Venture out beyond your normal shopping terrain and find out if there's a local farmers' market to browse. (Seems too drizzly to shop outside? Ask yourself, is a florescent-lit super market really more appealing?) It's a riot of competing shades of green. The recipes in this section include spinach, bok choy, and lots of fresh herbs, but load up on any green leaf that winks at you. A giant bundle of chard will serve several as a dinner side dish. Its cousin, kale, is a little hardier (but nutritionally super-powered), so pull out the tough stalks and use just the leaves. In both cases, wash well, steam lightly, and then flash sauté with garlic, olive oil, and a spritz of ume plum vinegar—delicious.

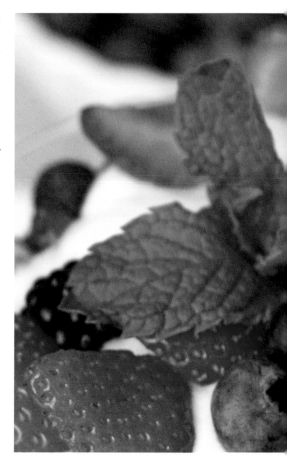

Color can also be your cooking teacher this season. When fresh foods change color over the heat, it's the signal they're done. Vegetables turn from dark green to bright green, as if their inner dimmer switch got turned up; salmon and shrimp go from translucent white-pink to a brighter orange-pink, and a white fish like black cod (it sounds like an oxymoron, but it really is white, and it's got great taste and texture) does an even subtler shift. It goes from milky opal to the chalky white of paint.

Organic yogurt is a worthwhile investment. Get the plain kind full of live active cultures and add the fruit yourself.

This is how you start to cook by instinct: your eye recognizes the moment something's done. In the case of fish, it means, please don't dawdle! Take the food off the heat right away. Few kitchen crimes are worse than overcooking a nice piece of fish, especially if you've invested in wild Alaskan salmon, which I recommend as it's usually lower in toxins, higher in nutrients, and less polluting to our environment. It's better to err on the side of caution and take the fish off early, put some foil over the pan, and let it steam itself to perfection for the last couple of minutes. The foods of spring are as new as the season, needing little manipulation or heat to bring out tender tastes. So it's best to handle with care, treating a nice ingredient like the newborn it is.

It's a delicate time for us, as well. We want to ease in to eating lighter because transitioning out of the dark takes time in humans, just as it takes time in nature. A soufflé, super easy to make, is a perfect springtime comfort food. The trick is in the flavors—if they're too muted, you'll be bored—so sniff out the most pungent basil and thyme you can find. An easy breakfast that is light yet substantial mixes yogurt and berries. Use plain, unsweetened yogurt that is full of active live cultures, like Stonyfield Farm, because these are essential for healthy digestion and most people are deficient in them. Thick Greek yogurt is another tasty option. Splurge on organic or at least rBGH-free. (Recombinant bovine growth hormone, a genetically engineered drug given to cows to increase productivity, is linked to rising cancer rates in humans.) Dairy can be surprisingly high in toxins, because they have a chance to ac-cumulate as they pass up the food chain from plant to animal and then on to you.

As I green my plate, I find new ways of greening my kitchen. Water and electricity have to come from somewhere, just like the food. I make an effort to use only what's needed. Each empty bottle is a candidate for reuse—millet and buckwheat find a home in clean tea caddies, while homemade marinades fill former mustard jars. The question that starts to drive my actions in the kitchen is, how little trash can I throw out this week?

Slowing down for just a second means the whole day can get greener. Lunch, snacks, and even dinner can be taken to work. I've fallen in love with my to-go eco kit: light steel containers that can be reused indefinitely. (They're great to bring leftovers home from restaurants as well.) I fill up my steel water canister—no more plastic bottles for me—and stash reusable utensils in my bag, happy that I'll never use plastic cutlery again. Small actions like these don't take much effort. They make me feel like a kid with a picnic; wherever I end up, I make the time to sit and eat quietly. And best of all I feel totally self-reliant, supplied with all I need to enjoy the spring day.

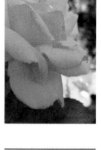

Spring is a time for setting new intentions.

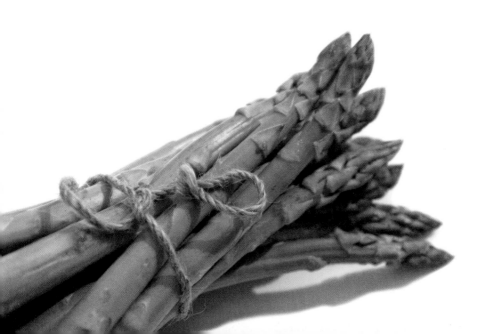

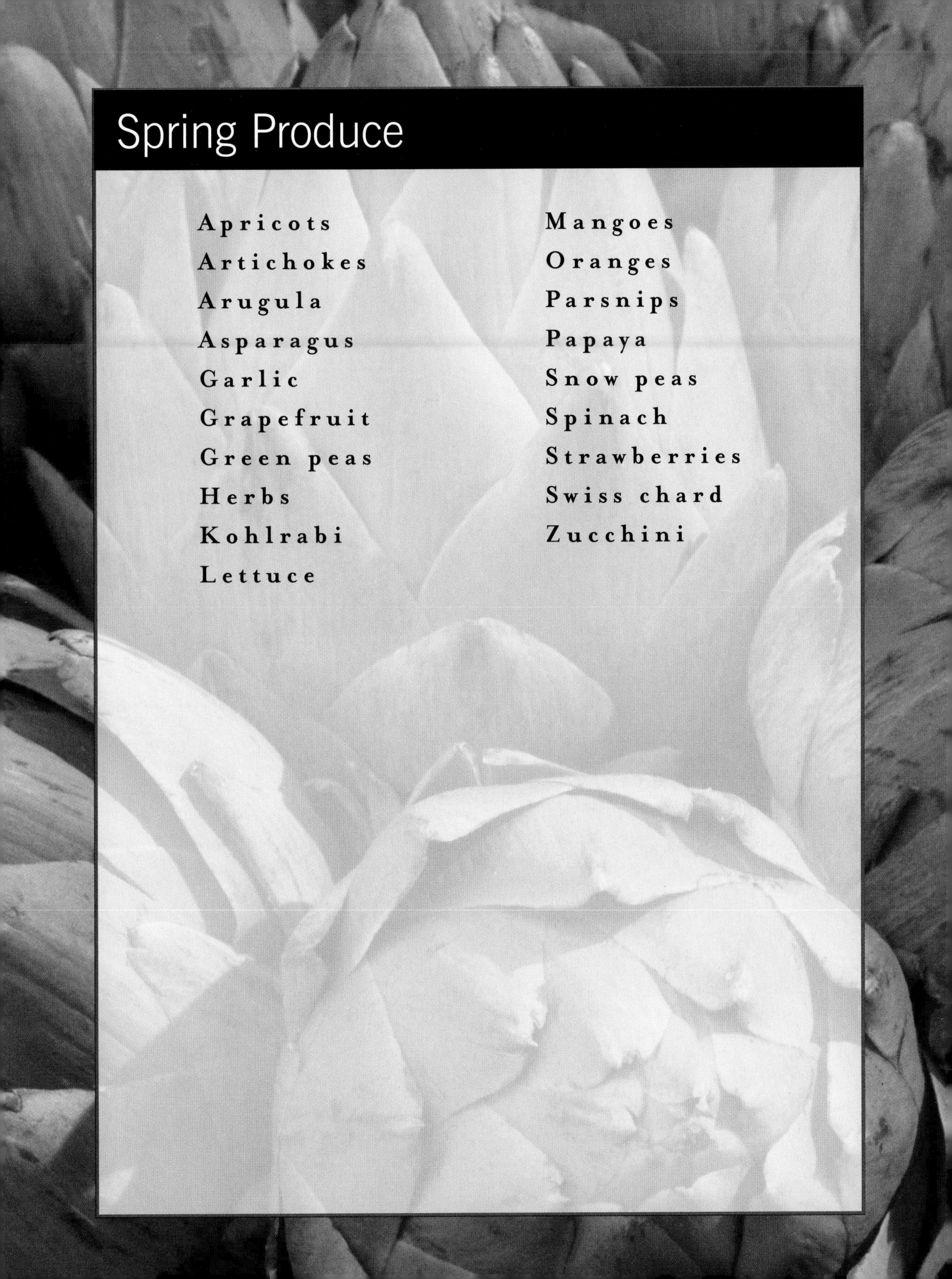

Spring Produce

Apricots

Artichokes

Arugula

Asparagus

Garlic

Grapefruit

Green peas

Herbs

Kohlrabi

Lettuce

Mangoes

Oranges

Parsnips

Papaya

Snow peas

Spinach

Strawberries

Swiss chard

Zucchini

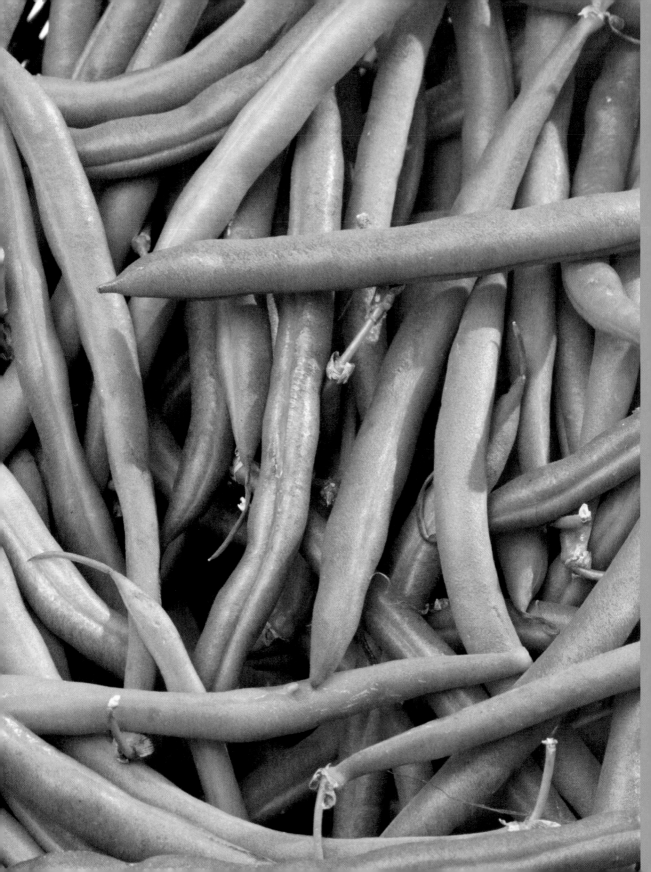

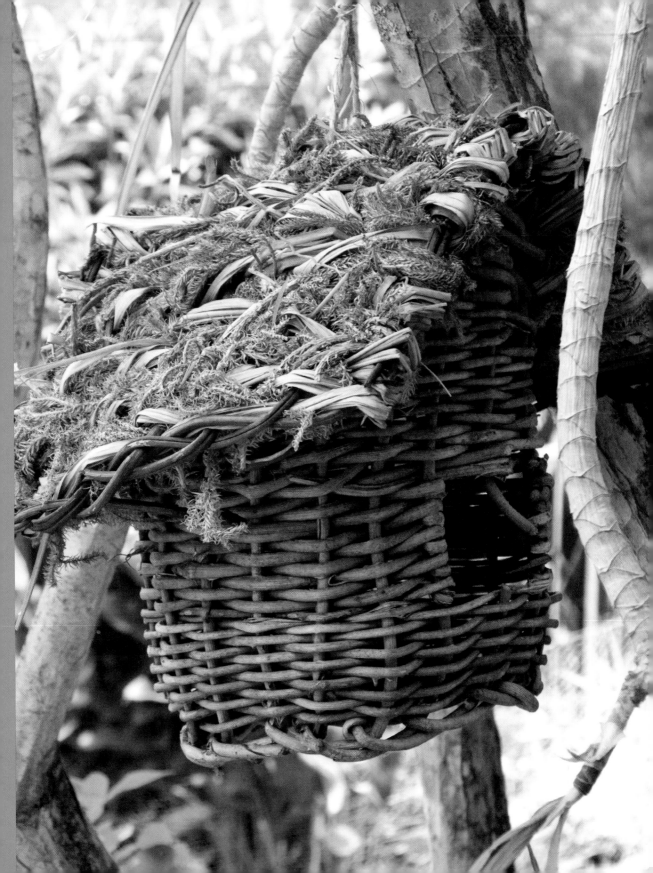

Yogurt and Berry Parfait

You can use
almost any
seasonal stone
fruit (peaches,
plums, apricots)
as a replacement
for the berries.
Adjust the amount
of Xylosweet used
depending how
sweet the fruit is.
You could also use
a couple layers
of crumbled
Blisscuits in this
recipe (similar to
a granola/yogurt/
berry parfait).

SERVES 2

1 cup sliced organic strawberries

2 cups seasonal organic blueberries

1 tablespoon Xylosweet

2 cups organic low-fat plain yogurt or goat's milk yogurt

I. Place strawberries and blueberries in a medium bowl. Gently toss with Xylosweet to coat. Allow to sit, refrigerated, for about 10 minutes.

2. Divide half the fruit between two parfait glasses or dessert bowls. Top each with ½ cup of yogurt, then another layer of berries and a final layer of yogurt. Serve immediately.

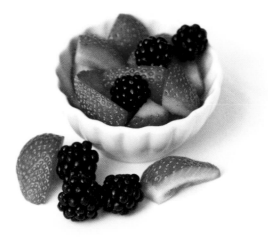

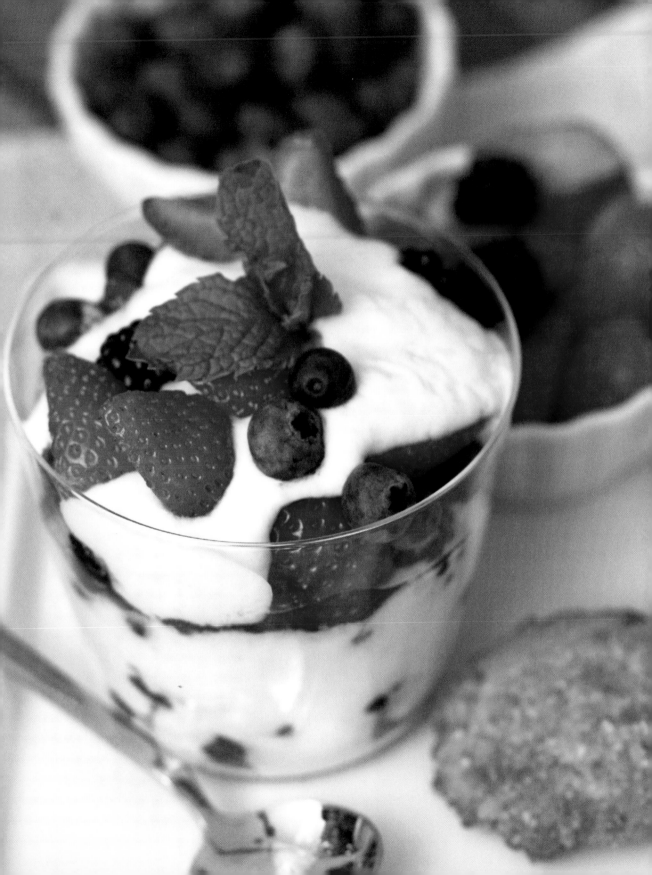

Jicama, Carrot, and Cucumber Salad with Citrus Dressing

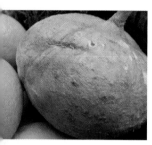

SERVES 4

Salad:

1 medium seedless cucumber, julienned

2 medium carrots, peeled and julienned

1 medium jicama, peeled and julienned

Creamy Curry-Citrus Dressing:

1 cup organic plain yogurt

1 small shallot, finely minced

1 teaspoon orange zest

2 tablespoons freshly squeezed orange juice

2 tablespoons freshly squeezed lemon juice

1 tablespoon extra virgin olive oil

½ teaspoon turmeric

⅛ teaspoon cayenne pepper, optional

Sea salt

Freshly-ground black pepper

Sprinkle salad with chopped toasted cashews or almonds, cilantro, or sulfite-free dried fruit such as apricots or golden raisins, or a combination of all three. Dressing can also be used as a dip for crudités.

1. Combine salad vegetables in a large mixing bowl. Cover and refrigerate until ready to serve.

2. Combine all dressing ingredients and whisk until thoroughly combined. Taste for

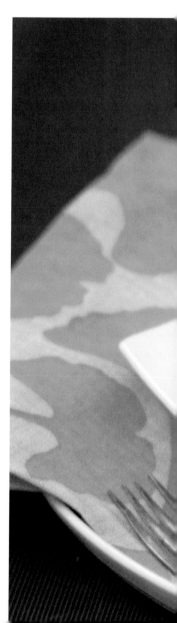

seasoning and add lemon juice or curry powder if desired. Salt and pepper to taste. Refrigerate until ready to serve.

3. Immediately before serving, add just enough dressing to coat salad vegetables lightly, and gently combine. Place vegetables on a serving platter or divide among individual serving dishes. Serve additional dressing on the side.

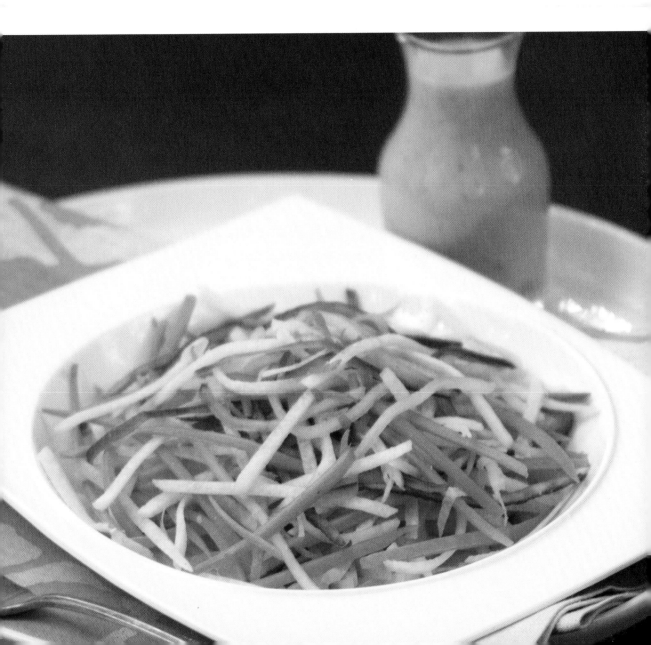

Herb Parmesan Soufflé

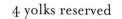

You can make this soufflé in one large soufflé pan—simply increase oven time to about 30 minutes or until soufflé has puffed and top has browned. As an alternative use goat's milk in place of whole milk.

2 ½ tablespoons unsalted butter, plus more
     for greasing ramekins

½ cup plus 3 tablespoons finely grated parmesan

3 tablespoons brown rice flour

1 cup organic whole milk, hot

½ teaspoon paprika

  Pinch of nutmeg

¼ teaspoon salt

  Freshly ground black pepper

¼ cup finely chopped fresh basil

2 teaspoons finely chopped fresh thyme

5 large eggs, divided, whites beaten to stiff peaks,
  4 yolks reserved

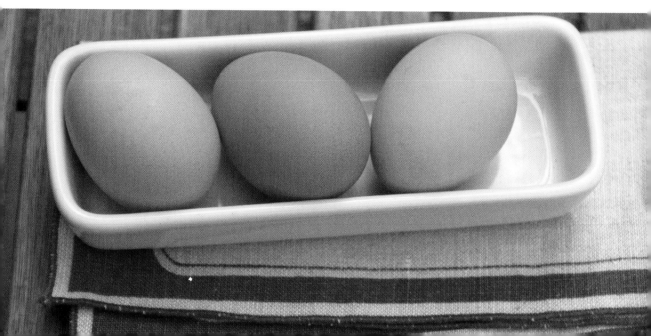

1. Preheat oven to 400°F.

2. Butter 8 (6-ounce) or 6 (8-ounce) individual ramekins. Coat with the 3 tablespoons parmesan and shake out any excess.

3. Place the 2 ½ tablespoons of butter and the flour in a medium-size heavy saucepan over medium heat. Cook, stirring constantly, until it begins to bubble. Remove from heat, let cool a few seconds, and then add hot milk all at once, whisking vigorously to blend.

4. Return to heat, whisking constantly, and bring to a simmer, cooking until mixture is fairly thick, about 3 minutes.

5. Whisk in the paprika, nutmeg, salt, pepper, basil, and thyme, and remove from heat.

6. Whisk in egg yolks one at a time. Set aside.

7. Whisk one-quarter of the egg whites into the cooked mixture. Fold the remaining three-quarters of the whites in rapidly, but delicately, and add in the remaining ½ cup parmesan as you fold. Pour batter into the prepared baking dishes.

8. Place ramekins on a sheet tray before placing in the oven. Reduce oven temperature to 375°F. Bake 20 minutes or until soufflés have puffed and tops are browned. Serve immediately.

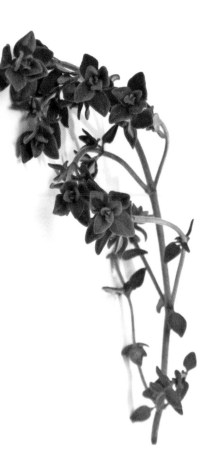

Grilled Shrimp Salad over Spinach

SERVES 4–6

Purchase shrimp from your local fish market or use a quality, already cooked, shelled, and deveined frozen brand.

- I pound jumbo shrimp, peeled and deveined
- I tablespoon coconut oil or olive oil
- Salt
- Freshly ground black pepper
- Pinch of cayenne pepper
- I teaspoon chopped fresh thyme
- I teaspoon chopped fresh rosemary
- 7 ounces baby spinach
- ⅓ cup Creamy Avocado Lime Dressing (pg. 50)

1. Heat a grill pan or skillet over high heat.
2. Toss shrimp with the oil, a bit of salt and pepper, cayenne, thyme, and rosemary. Skewer shrimp, add to pan, and cook for 2 minutes on each side or until just cooked through.
3. Toss spinach with dressing. Place in a shallow serving bowl and arrange shrimp on top.

As a variation, add a tablespoon of fresh chopped cilantro to the dressing.

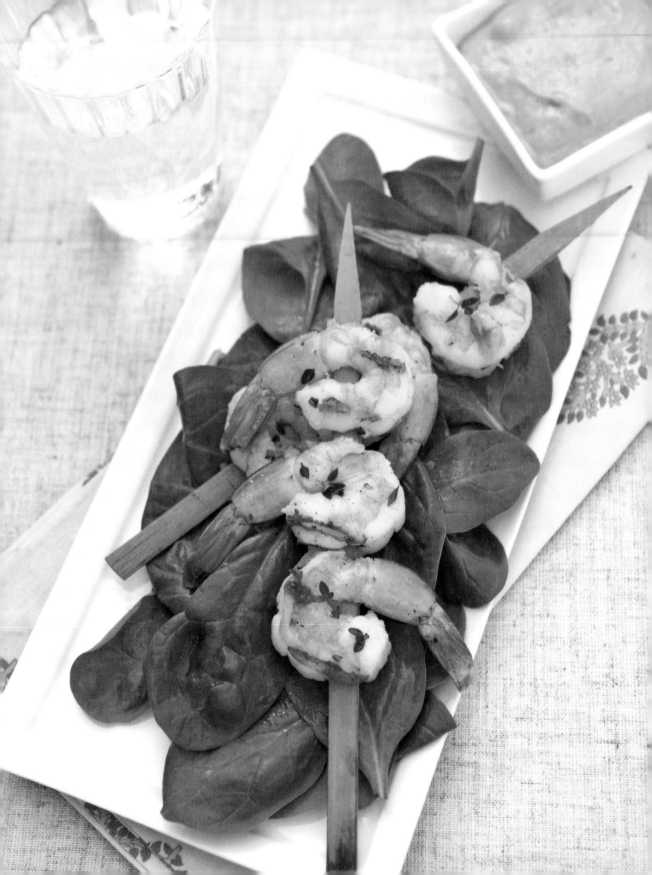

Living Wraps

SERVES 6

Check your local organic food store for soy wrappers, which are made from soy beans and come in a variety of colors. They are cholesterol- and fat-free and are an excellent source of protein.

1	teaspoon champagne vinegar
¼	teaspoon Xylosweet
½	teaspoon fresh lemon juice
2	tablespoons extra light olive oil
2–3	bunches (about 6 ounces) watercress
6	soy wrappers
1	red bell pepper, julienned
2	medium carrots, peeled and julienned
12	tiger shrimp, cooked

1. In a medium bowl, whisk together champagne vinegar, Xylosweet, lemon juice, and olive oil.

2. Add watercress to vinaigrette, tossing to coat.

3. Place soy papers on a clean work surface and fill each with a small amount of watercress mixture, julienned vegetables, and shrimp.

4. Beginning from one corner, wrap the paper into a cone shape. Wet seams at the end of soy wrapper to seal.

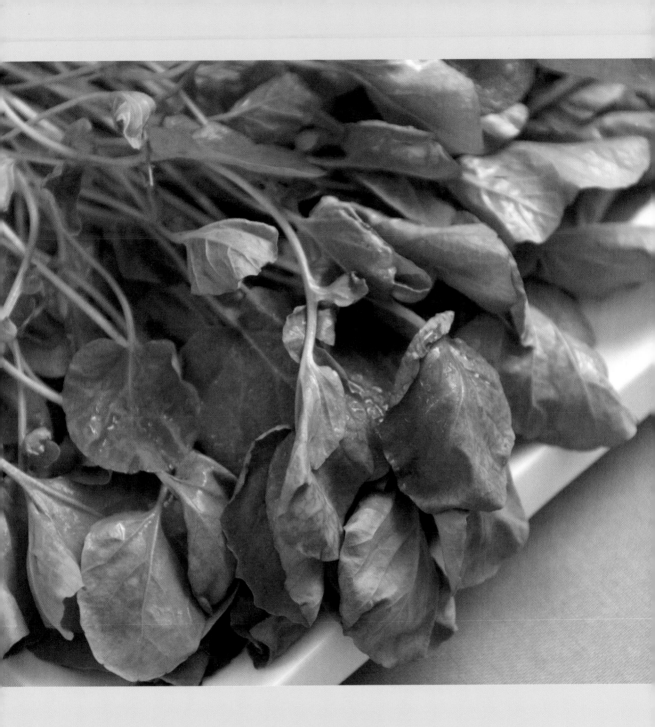

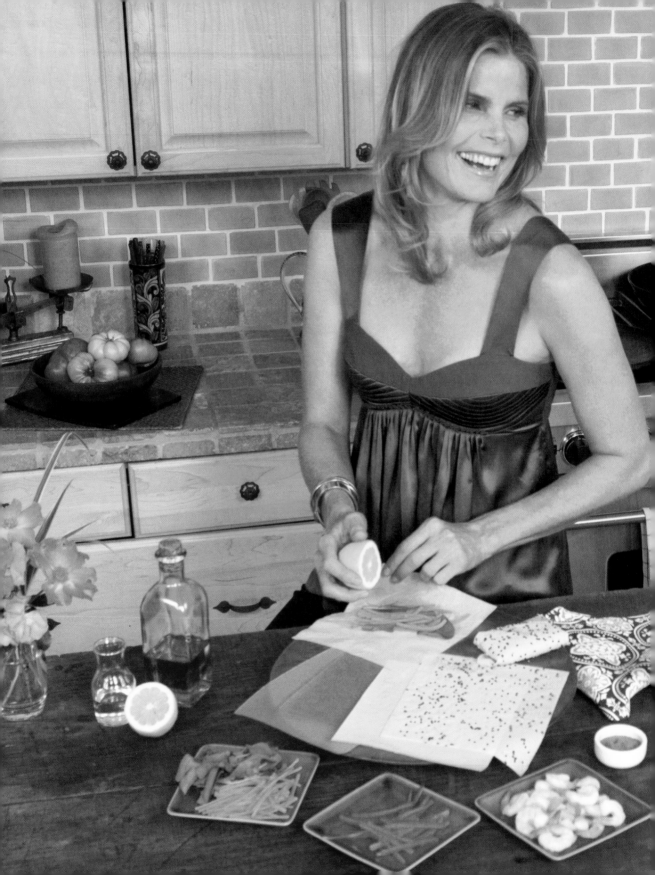

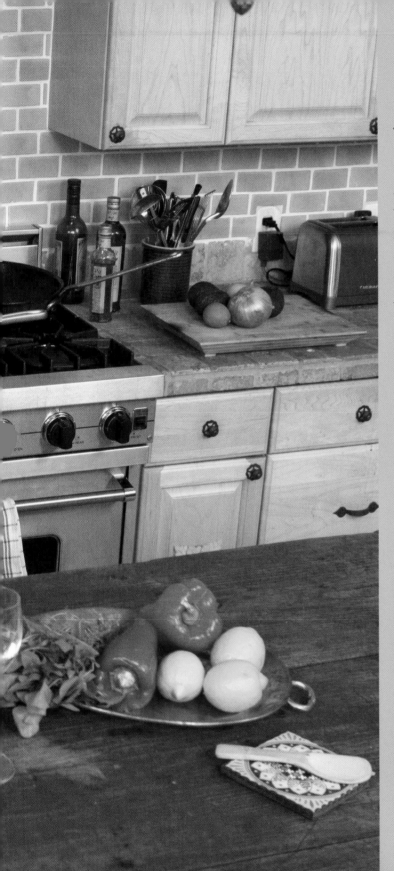

Rules that certain kinds of foods are for lunch, and others are for dinner, don't make sense to me. It's better for digestion to eat less at night, so when friends come over for a casual evening, I don't automatically load them down with heavy fare.

A wrap filled with fresh vegetables might find its way onto their dinner plate, with a colorful salad and some pureed soup from a bottomless tureen. I like to assemble some of the meal as we all hang out together, letting my guests tell me what extra ingredients they want to add to the mix and making sure hungrier guests get well satisfied. Food becomes more fun when it's a group effort.

Almond and Garlic–Crusted Chicken Breasts

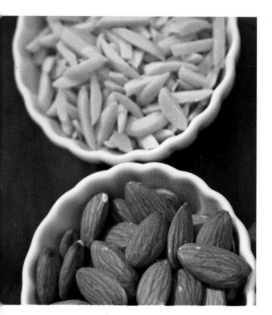

SERVES 4

½ cup sliced almonds

½ cup almond meal

4 cloves garlic, chopped

2 tablespoons chopped flat-leaf parsley

1 whole egg

4 (6-ounce) boneless, skinless, organic free-range chicken breasts

Salt

Pepper

2 teaspoons coconut oil

You can substitute the almonds with other nuts you may have on hand, such as pine nuts, hazelnuts, or pecans. Serve with a side salad.

1. Combine almonds, almond meal, garlic, and parsley in the work bowl of a food processor and pulse 3 or 4 times to combine.

2. Place egg in a large shallow bowl or pie plate and beat briefly with a fork.

3. Place almond mixture in a separate shallow bowl.

4. Pat chicken dry and season both sides with salt and pepper.

5. Dip chicken into egg, and then press into nut mixture to coat on all sides.

6. Place chicken on a baking sheet, cover, and refrigerate for at least 20 minutes to set the crust.

7. Preheat oven to 350°F.

8. Heat oil in a large skillet over medium heat. Add chicken and cook until the crust turns golden brown, 3 to 4 minutes per side.

9. Place chicken in a baking dish and cook until an instant-read thermometer registers an internal temperature of 160°F, about 15 minutes.

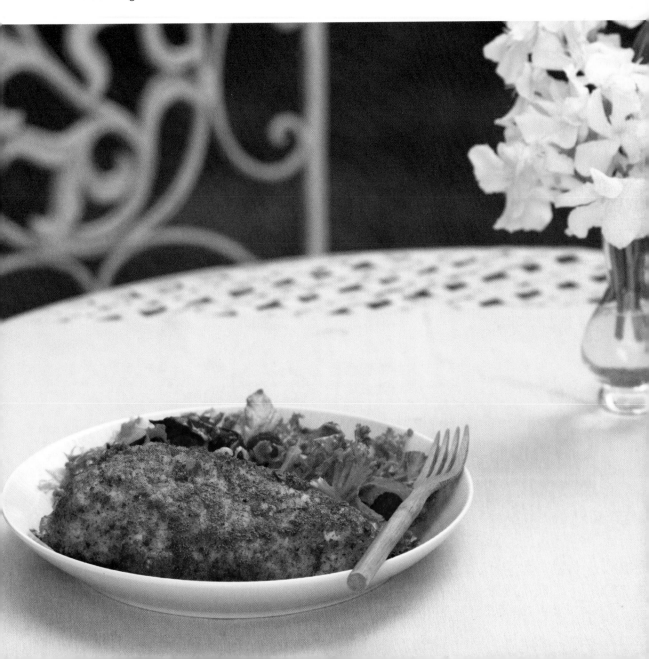

Roasted Artichoke, Eggplant, and Tomato Stacks

SERVES 4

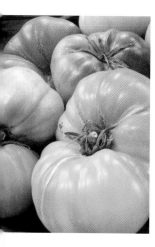

1 large organic lemon, juiced (about ½ cup)

4 fresh, whole organic artichokes, about 3–4 inches in diameter

1 large organic eggplant, about 3 inches diameter, unpeeled

2 large organic tomatoes (preferably heirloom), about 3–4 inches diameter

3 tablespoons coconut or olive oil

Sea salt

Freshly ground black pepper

1 tablespoon fresh thyme, plus extra for garnish

1. Preheat oven to 400°F.

2. Fill a large bowl with cold water and the lemon juice.

3. Remove all leaves from artichokes. Cut off bottom stem so artichoke heart will sit flat on the baking sheet. Remove the inner fuzzy choke (a melon ball tool works great for this) and any small prickly leaves. Place the artichokes in the lemon water as you finish peeling and preparing each one and while you are preparing the eggplant and tomatoes.

4. Cut eggplant width-wise into rounds about ½ inch thick. You should have at least 8 rounds. Place on a baking sheet lined with aluminum foil.

5. Cut the tomatoes width-wise into rounds about ½ inch thick. Again, you should have at least 8 rounds. Place on the baking sheet with the eggplant slices.

6. Remove artichokes from water and pat dry. Place them on the tray with tomatoes and eggplant.

7. Using a pastry brush, brush eggplant, tomato, and artichokes on both sides with about 2 tablespoons of oil. Season both sides with salt, pepper, and a sprinkle of thyme.

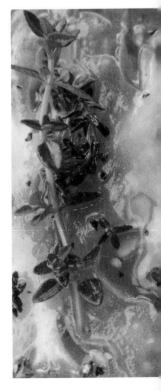

8. Place tray in the preheated oven and bake, gently turning vegetables once, until artichoke hearts are tender when pierced with a fork and eggplant and tomatoes are tender and beginning to caramelize, about 30 minutes. Remove from oven and tent with foil to keep warm.

9. To serve, place 1 artichoke heart (stem-end down) on each of four individual serving plates. Alternate stacking them with 1 slice of eggplant and 1 slice of tomato. Each stack should end up having about 2 each of eggplant and tomato slices. Finish with a drizzle of oil and garnish with a sprig of fresh thyme if desired.

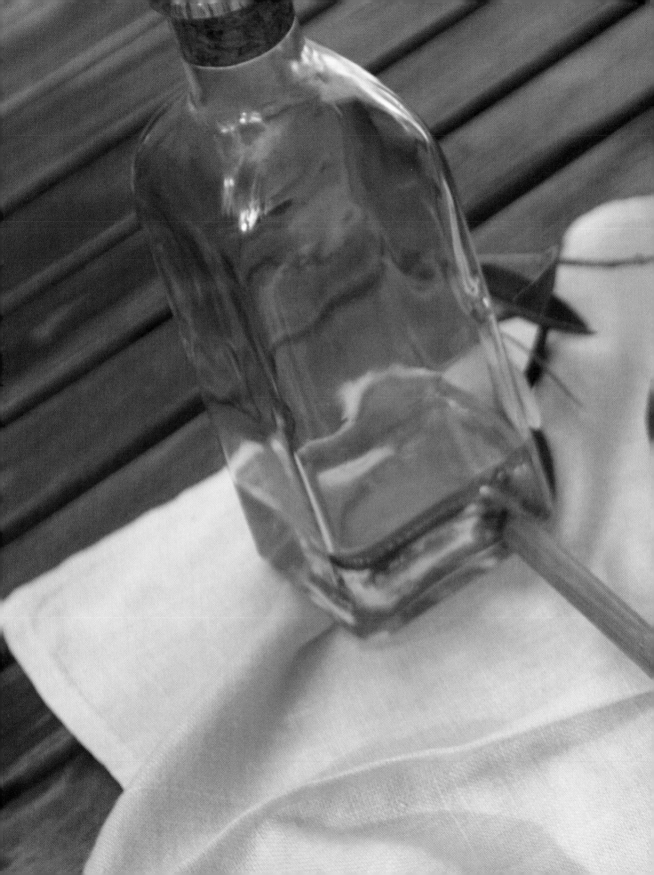

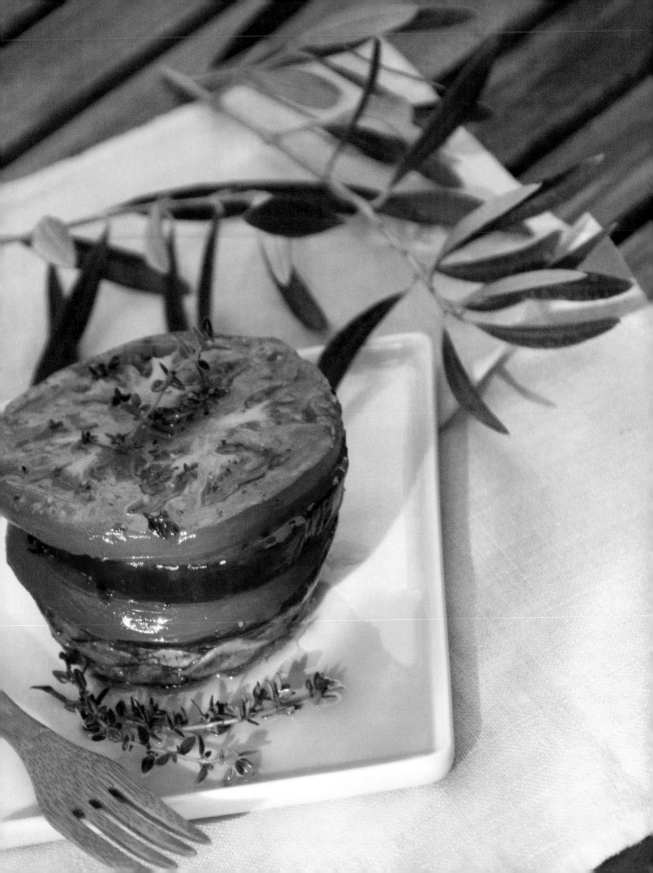

Seared Wild Salmon with Minted Mango Salsa

This salsa would also be delicious served with the Vietnamese Chicken Lettuce Wraps with Mint-Basil Sauce (pg. 120).

SERVES 4

Mango Salsa:

- 1 medium, ripe mango, peeled and diced
- 1 cup diced English hothouse cucumber
- 2 green onions, sliced
- 1 medium tomato, seeds removed and diced
- 1 small jalapeño, seeded, finely minced, optional
- 1 clove garlic, finely minced
- 1 tablespoon coarsely chopped mint
- 2 tablespoons fresh lime juice
  Sea salt

Wild Salmon:

- 2 tablespoons coconut or olive oil
- 4 (4- to 5-ounce) wild salmon fillets
  Freshly ground black pepper

1. Combine mango, cucumber, green onions, tomato, jalapeño, garlic, mint, and lime juice in a medium bowl, stirring gently to combine. Add salt to taste. Cover and set aside. If not using right away, salsa can be chilled for up to 6 hours.

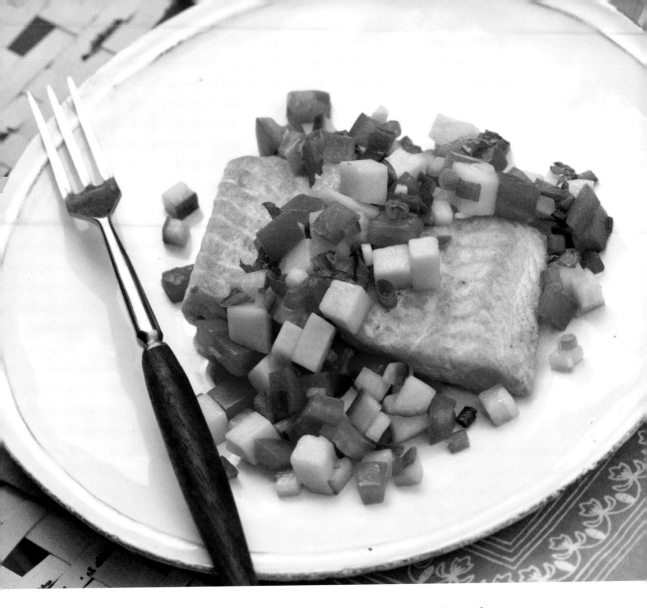

2. Season salmon fillets on both sides with salt and pepper. Heat oil
   in a large, heavy skillet over medium heat. Sear salmon on both
   sides until golden brown and flakey, about 3 minutes each side.
   Spoon salsa on top and serve immediately.

Roasted Bok Choy and Cauliflower with Cumin and Mint

SERVES 4

Bok Choy and Cauliflower:

- 2 medium, fresh organic bok choy (about 2 pounds)
- 2 tablespoons coconut or olive oil
  Sea salt
  Freshly ground black pepper
- 2 cups cauliflower florets

Vinaigrette:

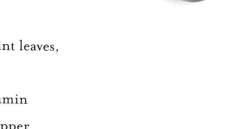

- ¼ cup olive oil
- 3 tablespoons freshly squeezed organic lemon juice
- ½ teaspoon lemon zest
- 2 tablespoons fresh mint leaves, coarsely chopped
- 1 ½ teaspoons ground cumin
- ⅛ teaspoon cayenne pepper
  Sea salt
  Freshly ground black pepper

1. Preheat oven to 400°F.
2. Cut bok choy in half length-wise and place on a baking sheet lined with aluminum foil. Drizzle with 1 tablespoon of the coconut oil and sprinkle with salt and pepper.

3. Place cauliflower florets on another foiled baking sheet. Drizzle with the remaining tablespoon coconut oil and sprinkle with salt and pepper.

4. Place both trays in the preheated oven and bake, turning and alternating racks once, until vegetables are tender when pierced with a fork, about 20 minutes. When done, remove from oven and cover with aluminum foil to keep warm.

5. While vegetables are roasting, prepare vinaigrette. In a small bowl combine the olive oil, lemon juice, lemon zest, mint, cumin, and cayenne pepper. Season with salt and pepper if desired. Set aside until vegetables are roasted.

6. While still warm, remove bok choy and cauliflower from baking sheet and chop into 1-inch pieces and place in a large bowl. Dress vegetables with vinaigrette and mix gently to combine. Place vegetables on serving platter or divide among individual serving dishes. Garnish with a sprig of mint if desired.

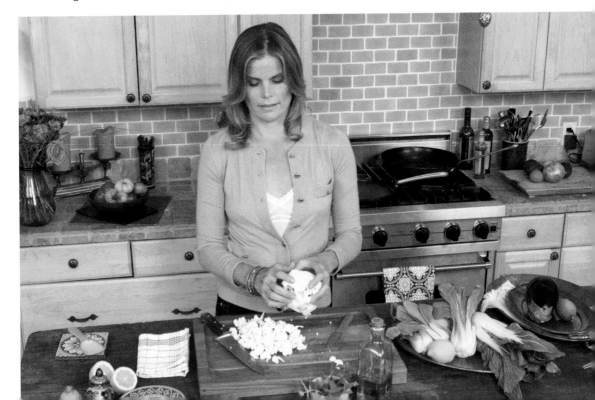

Black Cod with Snow Peas

If you aren't able
to find black
cod (also known
as sablefish or
butterfish) you
could substitute
your favorite
white fish.

SERVES 4

4 (4-ounce) black cod fillets, about ½-inch thick,
skin removed

¾ cup All-Purpose Marinade (pg. 49)

1 pound Chinese snow peas

1 cup fresh organic orange juice

1 (1-inch) piece fresh ginger, peeled and sliced

1 tablespoon unsalted butter

Sea salt

Freshly ground black pepper

1 tablespoon coconut or olive oil

1. Place fillets in a nonreactive container or large plastic
bag and add half the marinade, reserving the other half.
Seal container and refrigerate for about 20 minutes.

2. Meanwhile, bring a large pot of salted water to a boil.
Add snow peas and cook for 30 seconds. Immediately
drain under cold running water. Set aside.

3. To make sauce, place reserved marinade, orange juice, and ginger
into a small saucepan over medium heat. Simmer until liquid
begins to thicken, about 4 minutes. Remove from heat and
discard ginger. Stir in butter. Season with salt and pepper.
Cover to keep warm, and set aside.

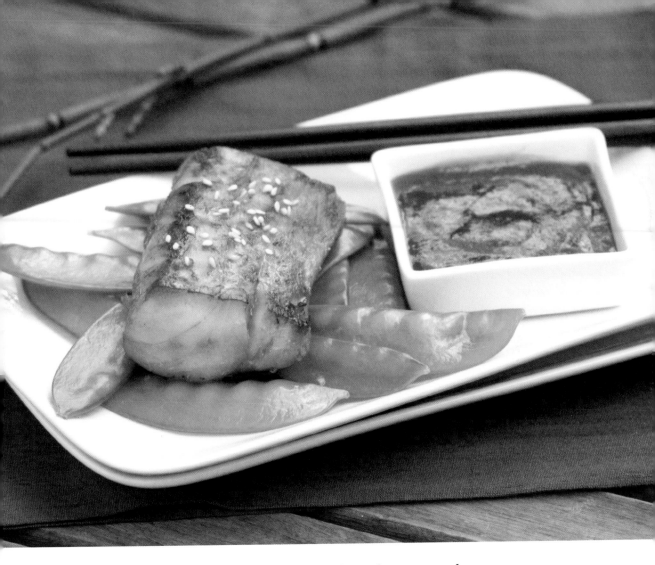

4. Remove fillets from marinade and pat dry with paper towels. Season both sides with salt and pepper. Heat coconut oil in a large skillet. Sear fillets on each side until they are golden, being careful not to overcook, about 3 minutes on each side.

5. To serve, divide snow peas between four dinner plates, top with a fillet, and spoon a little sauce over the top. Serve any additional sauce on the side.

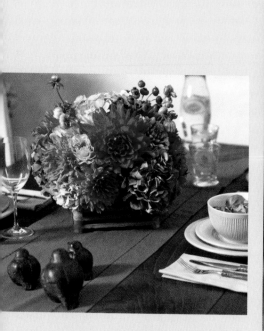

Now more than ever, we need to get back to communal eating. With family, with old friends, or new acquaintances—sharing food is the best way I know to make true human connection. It can be incredibly simple: a couple of simple dishes and one or two decorations is enough. No one expects perfection. As families get more fragmented and we live more isolated lives, eating together is meaningful and rewarding.

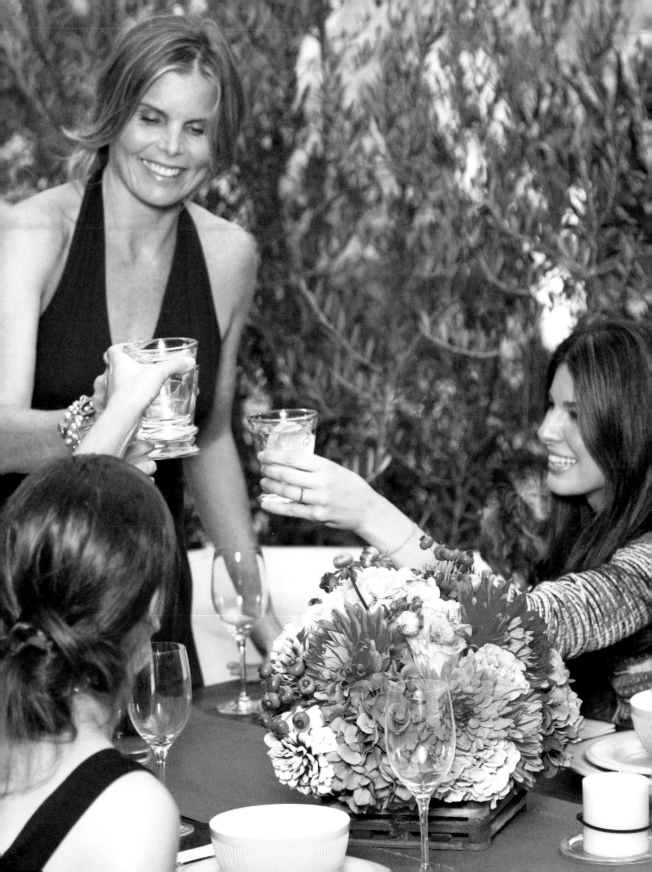

Ricotta "No Bread" Pudding with Blueberries

SERVES 6–8

Substitute any fresh, organic seasonal fruit for the blueberries. As an alternative, you can use goat's or sheep's milk ricotta in place of the part skim milk ricotta.

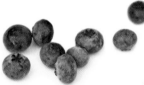

Coconut oil for greasing pan

1 tablespoon ground almond meal,
plus more for coating ramekins

1 pound fresh, organic, part skim milk ricotta

5 large egg yolks

¼ cup Xylosweet

Pinch of sea salt

1 teaspoon grated lemon zest

5 large egg whites, beaten to stiff peaks

1 cup organic blueberries for garnish

1. Preheat oven to 375°F.

2. Grease an 8-inch square baking pan. Sprinkle with a little almond meal, shaking pan to coat.

3. In a medium bowl, combine the ricotta with the egg yolks, the remaining tablespoon almond meal, Xylosweet, salt, and lemon zest. Mix well to combine. Gently fold in the egg whites.

4. Pour mixture into prepared pan. Bake for about 25 minutes or until center is slightly jiggly and top is lightly browned. Turn off heat and leave in oven for an additional 5 minutes. Remove from oven. Serve warm or at room temperature topped with fresh blueberries. Refrigerate leftovers.

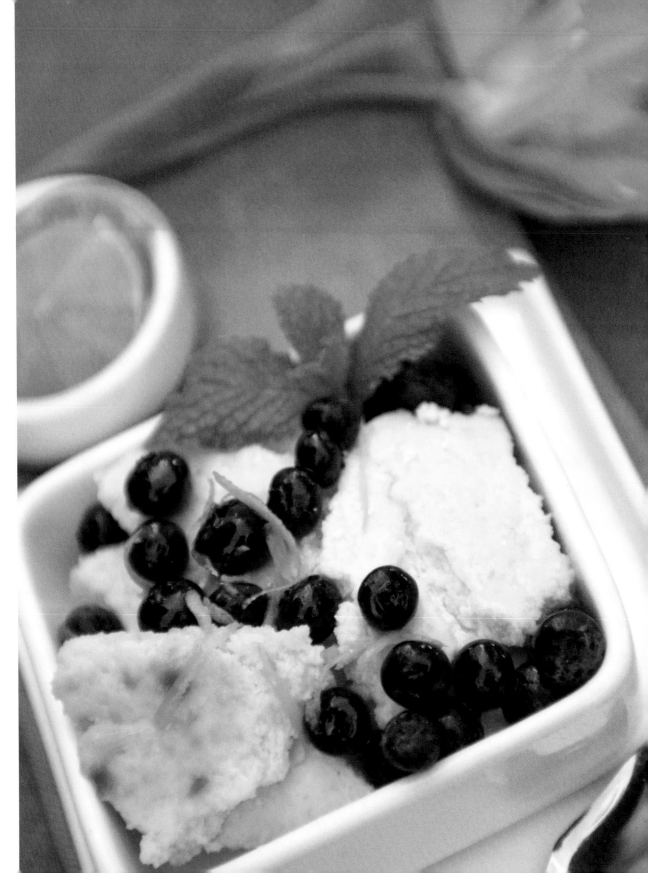

Apple Walnut Blisscuit Bars

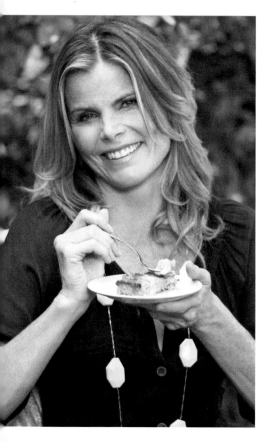

Stir a half cup of any kind of chopped dried fruit into the batter before baking.

MAKES 8 BARS

4 cups Basic Blisscuit dough (pg. 36)

2 gala apples, peeled, cored, and chopped into ½-inch cubes

2 tablespoons lemon juice

1 ½ tablespoons ground cinnamon

2 tablespoons coconut flour

¾ cup unsweetened organic applesauce

¼ cup chopped walnuts

1. Preheat oven to 325°F. Cover an 8-inch square baking dish with parchment paper and set aside.

2. Place chopped apples into a bowl and toss with lemon juice, ground cinnamon, and coconut flour. Set aside.

3. Stir applesauce and walnuts into the Blisscuit dough until thoroughly combined.

4. Fold apple mixture into the dough and spoon batter into prepared baking dish.

5. Bake for 15 to 20 minutes or until the top is golden brown. Let cool before cutting.

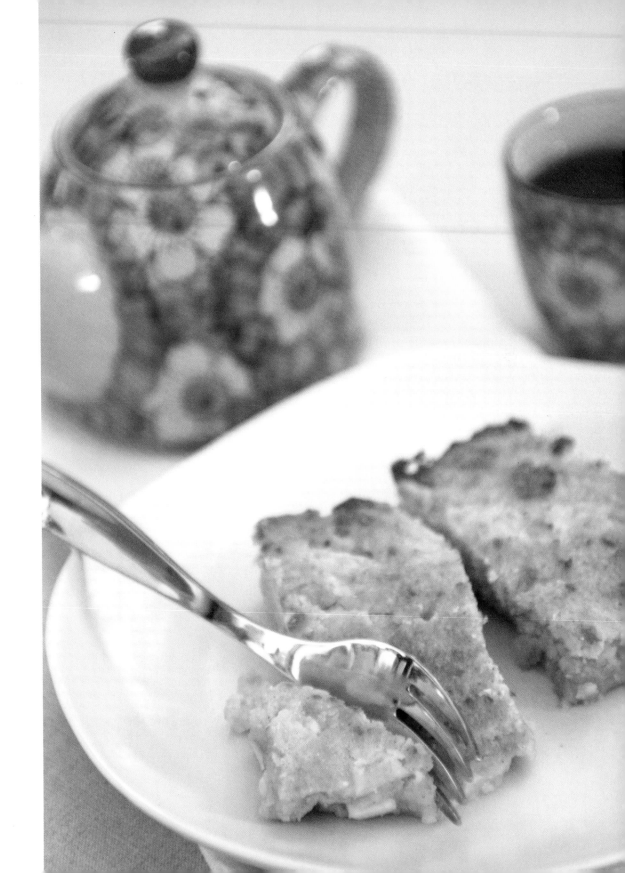

Zucchini Walnut Dip

This dip is great
with crudités
of celery and
cauliflower or
toasted whole
wheat pita bread.

This dip can be
served warm,
at room
temperature,
or chilled. Dip
can be made up
to 3 days before
eaten if kept
refrigerated
in an airtight
container.
Serve with
Quinoa Millet
Crackers
(pg. 94).

MAKES 2 CUPS

2   medium zucchini, sliced

2   tablespoons olive oil

¼   cup chopped red onion

½   cup plain organic yogurt or goat's milk yogurt

1   tablespoon lemon juice

1   clove garlic

½   teaspoon paprika

    Sea salt

¼   cup whole walnuts

1. Place zucchini in a microwave-safe bowl, cover with plastic wrap, and heat on high for 1 minute or until cooked through.

2. Place oil, onion, yogurt, lemon juice, garlice, paprika, salt, and walnuts along with the zucchini in the work bowl of a food processor or blender and process until evenly ground but still a little chunky.

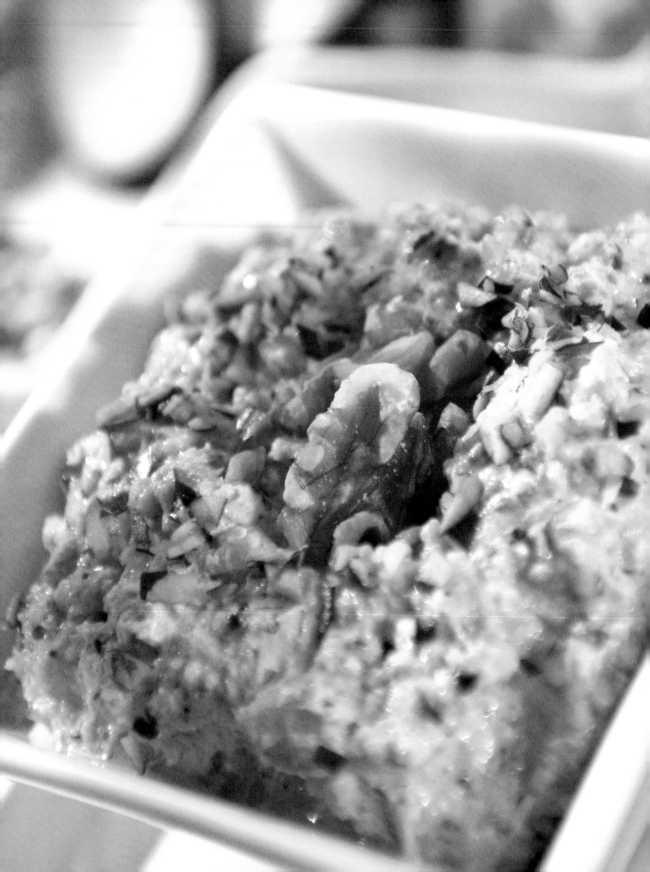

Quinoa Millet Crackers

SERVES 6

¾	cup coarse ground quinoa
¾	cup coarse ground millet
3	tablespoons coconut oil or olive oil
2	tablespoons honey
5	tablespoons water
1	large egg white
1 ½	teaspoons salt

1. Preheat oven to 325°F. Line a baking sheet with parchment paper.

2. Mix quinoa and millet together in a small bowl.

3. In a medium bowl, mix together oil, honey, water, egg white, and salt.

4. Add millet mixture to oil mixture ⅓ cup at a time, stirring to incorporate after each addition, until a rough dough begins to form (the dough should have the consistency of a very thick batter).

5. Knead the dough for about 2 minutes, adding additional quinoa and millet if dough is very sticky, or water if it becomes crumbly. Place dough on prepared baking sheet and, using a rolling pin, roll out to about ¼ inch thick.

6. Using a small, sharp knife, cut dough into 1-inch squares.

7. Bake for 25 to 30 minutes or until crackers are golden brown and crispy.
8. Allow crackers to sit for 15 to 20 minutes before breaking apart.

Roasted Red Bell Pepper Tapenade

SERVES 6–8

1 ¼ cups roasted red bell peppers

⅓ cup extra light olive oil

¼ cup pine nuts, toasted

¼ cup flat-leaf parsley, stems removed

Toasting the pine nuts adds a deliciously nutty taste to this tapenade. Lighten this recipe with a half cup of vegetable broth to make a colorful sauce for fish or pasta.

1. Place all ingredients into a blender or food processor.
2. Pulse until ingredients are combined but still a bit chunky.
3. Chill in the refrigerator until ready to use.

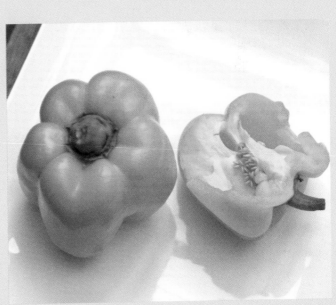

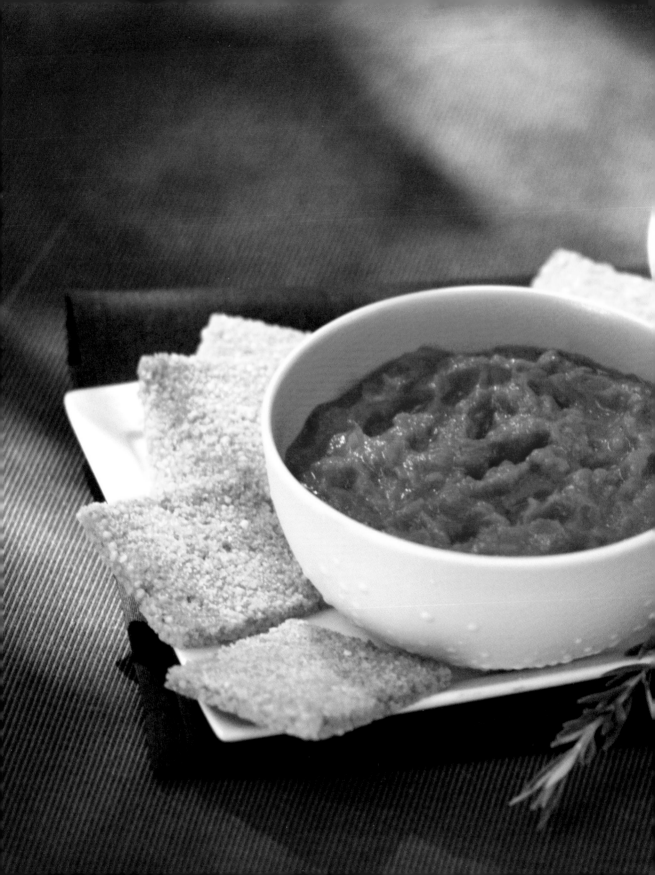

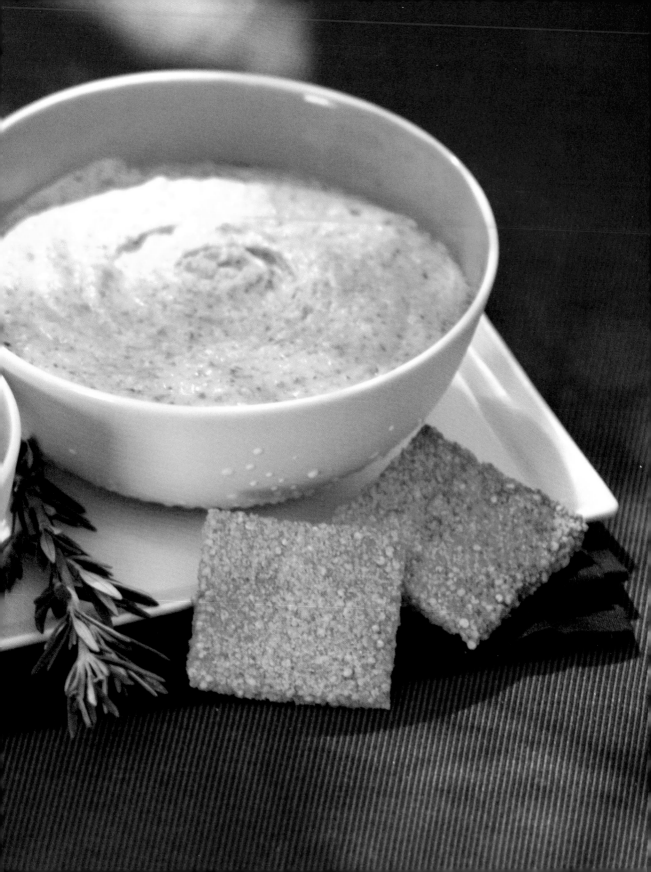

The Green Kitchen Challenge

Sustainability starts with the most essential part of life, eating. I created an earth-friendly kitchen by challenging myself to make one small change a week to my regular routine. (See the Resources section for products.)

1 I committed to breaking one bad habit per week: **Turn off taps when normally they'd be running; set up a streamlined recycling system by devoting a clean receptacle to non-landfill trash, unplug appliances when not in use because they steal energy for no good reason. (I even tied a ribbon around the faucet to remind me of my promise.)**

2 I determined to cut solid waste in half. **I deemed plastic containers, Ziploc bags, and glass jars non-disposable items and reused them unless they'd stored raw meats or fish. A small bag-drying rack on the counter top is a godsend for repurposing bags. Fifteen** minutes spent organizing container drawers so each item has a lid pays off. I put a selection of these items in my car with my cloth shopping totes to use at markets and salad bars.

3 I made a decision to buy bulk items whenever possible so I could take my own containers. **Beans, pulses, nuts, baking ingredients, and whatever grains you use can be purchased this way, and it usually works out cheaper than brand-name goods.**

4 I pledged to not throw away food, and to cook or freeze whatever had just lost freshness. **Soft vegetables**

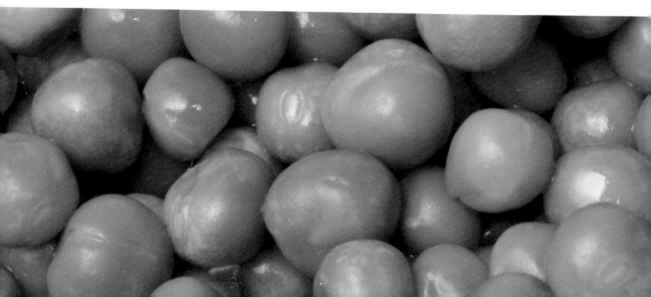

can easily become a vegetable stock for soups; overripe tomatoes become sauce; bananas and other fruit going mushy can get frozen in chunks for smoothies. Half a loaf of bread can be sliced and frozen on purchase. Woody herbs like rosemary and thyme can be dried; leafy ones like cilantro get pureed and frozen in ice-cube trays for later use. Our grandmothers did it—why can't we?

5 I went cold-turkey on toxic, chemical-filled cleaning products. **There's no need to buy an armory of new stuff, as an all-purpose green cleaner covers many needs. Reusable cleaning materials like micro-fiber dusting cloths and old-fashioned dishtowels mean that (recycled) paper towels are saved for true one-time use.**

6 I installed a good water filter for my drinking, cooking, and vegetable-washing needs. **This costs some money up front but delivers pure water free of chemicals and contaminants, without the** environmental impact of bottled water production and delivery. I fill up a metal canister to take water with me when I leave.

7 I put a large container outside my door to gather rainwater for plants and pets. **It's a small act of conservation, but it feels great to scoop water up and bring it inside—children learn from it, too.**

8 I invested in some solar panels for my roof to lessen my reliance on nonrenewable resources. **The amount of energy I saved surprised me; the initial investment paid off quicker than I'd thought.**

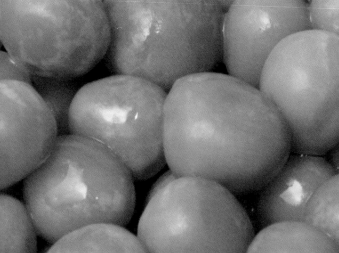

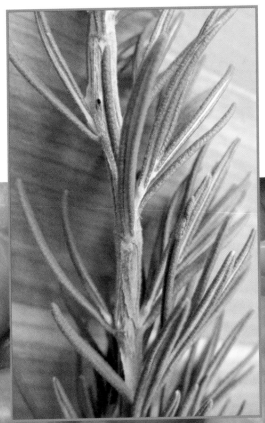

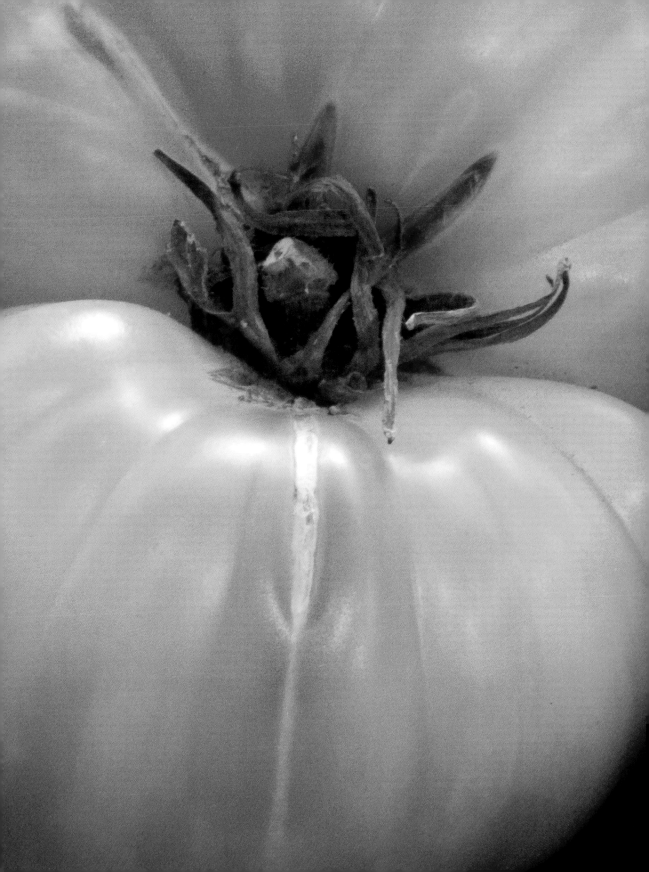

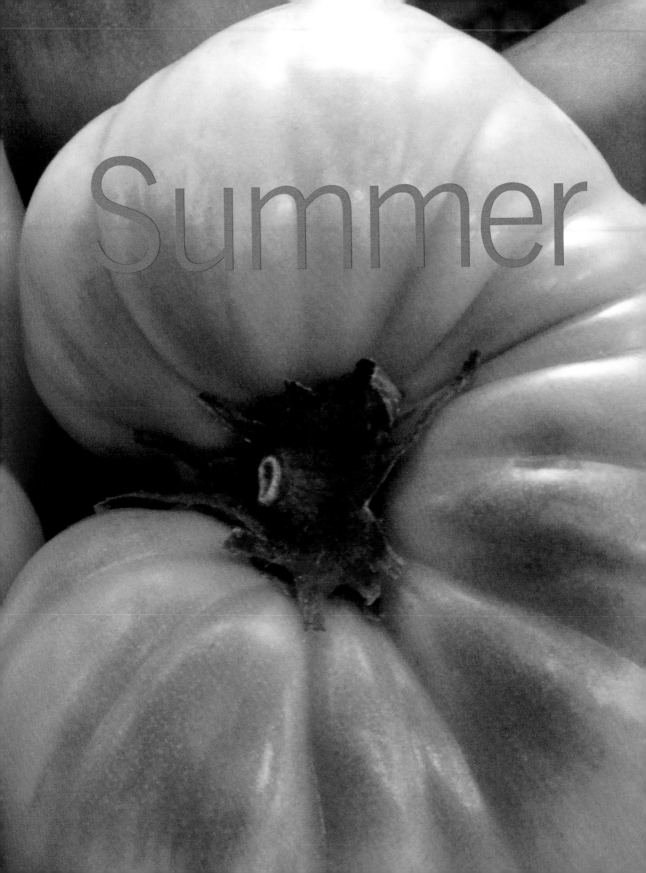

Summer

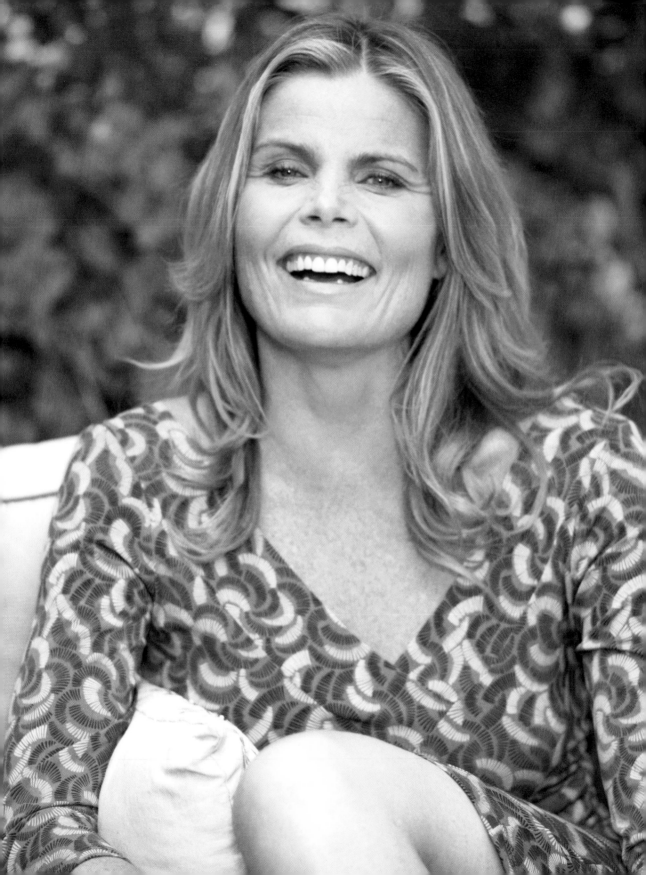

Plunge into Bold Flavors

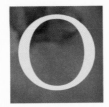f all the four seasons, summer is the one my senses love the most. Maybe it's because I'm a nature girl at heart; I love to cook—and eat—with my hands, ideally outside. Summer gives full license for that kind of thing. It practically begs you to get physical with your food—pulling fat berries off brambles or twisting plump tomatoes off the vine. You can plunge your clean hands into salad to give it a toss, and then eat chicken with your fingers as you sit outdoors with friends. Even if you're nowhere near a wild berry patch (or find hands-on cooking too sloppy), the piles of produce on sale are asking to be touched. Take more time than usual to select, sniff, and squeeze what you buy—the hot-weather months are when food gets truly sensual.

The things I like to make in summer are full of gutsy flavor. I adore ingredients that announce they've just come from the earth. Watercress pops with peppery spice; its cousin, arugula, has a similar bite. With these on a plate, and a fantastic oil, I'm halfway to heaven. Fennel, another spicy plant with an aniseed scent, may be a new addition to your kitchen. It lends a hint of French country cooking to two dishes here, scallops and halibut, and once you get to know it, fennel will be your friend. In cooked dishes or shaved raw onto salads, it greatly expands your collection of fresh-food flavors. Giant heirloom tomatoes, when married to garlic and a bit of jalapeño, make a cold gazpacho that is (harmlessly!) addicting. It's so good, many have been known to finish it for breakfast with a dollop of yogurt and a sprinkle of savory seeds. Stir in avocado, and you have a filling lunch.

Don't forget herbs, those often-overlooked details that should actually be the first stop. Grow your own basil—a surprisingly easy feat, even if you just buy a big pot from the grocer and keep it going on the windowsill—and you can have all-season access to fresh-made pesto, one of man's, or probably woman's, greatest inventions that miraculously tastes delicious on pretty much everything. I've used it here on the Pesto Halibut with Braised Fennel. I often pair it with heirloom tomatoes or put it on an endive salad with a few crushed walnuts for a quick side dish.

Summer's also a time for more sharing, with less ceremony. When everyone's barefoot, entertaining seems easier. For one thing it's simple for guests to contribute—one brings asparagus, another brings peaches, and you provide the fresh crab claws and

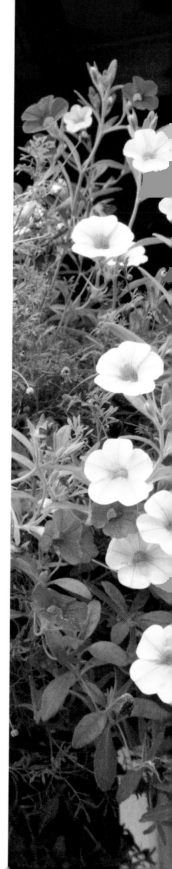

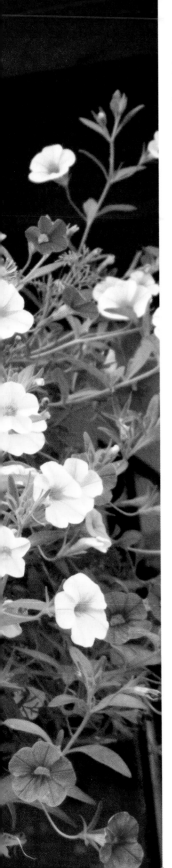

homemade mayonnaise. Before you know it, the meal's done. All you have to do is lay out paper towels and—presto! Nobody expects a matching set of anything when the lingering sunset is the big event. Kids and adults alike love the Oven "Fried" Chicken, a healthy version of a hot-weather favorite. Pair it with Baked Sweet Potato Sticks and Sugar-Free Ketchup to win extra points, and then ask someone else to shuck corn on the cob. Bring out the homemade raspberry dressing or the creamy ranch substitute made with tofu, served in a nice pourer for the table, and even prewashed, precut salad will taste sensational.

If you've got time, round out your table with portobello mushrooms, a food that's unfairly considered a vegetarian meal, as if omnivores won't love their rich flavor too. They should be rediscovered: when you're on your own, they're satisfying as a lighter dinner with a side of your choice, and so easy to make. The secret is to make sure they're fresh. Check that the gills on the underside are firm, not mushy.

And then there's the fruit! For years I ate almost no fruit, such was my allegiance to a low-fructose diet. It worked for me then, but now I'm easing up. The succulent pleasures of ripe fruits in season are too good for the soul to pass up. I don't sugar them or douse them in cream, however; I love my summer fruits in ultra-simple recipes like soufflés that are—just like those peach pies of my youth—a joy to eat.

That's what eating this season should be about: fun. There's something about cooking on a warm evening—with the windows open and the radio on—that causes you to think, this is my passion!

Not just my duty. You're more likely to experiment, mixing colors on the plate, reaching for a new kind of oil to drizzle on your leaves, and tearing up some herbs that may or may not work. In this way, each one of us becomes an artist, connecting to that creativity that's always there within, yet sometimes silenced in the rush of daily life. It's as simple as selecting yellow squash to offset the hue of red peppers, then cutting them up in artful new shapes and sprinkling a final note of Italian parsley for a full spectrum of color. Or presenting a meal in picturesque dishes, making a choice about each serving spoon. Many years of cooking simple food has shown me that I don't have to be a painter or sculptor to make meaningful art. What's on my plate is my own happy creation.

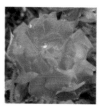

It's hard to go wrong in summer if you mix juicy vegetables on a plate. Just let your taste buds be your guide.

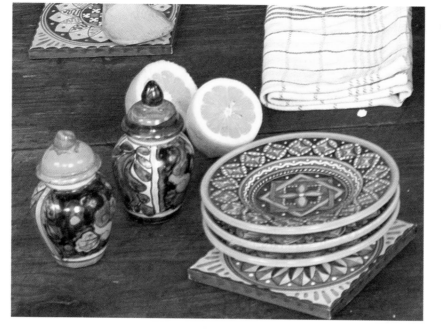

Summer Produce

Apricots

Basil

Berries: strawberries, black raspberries, blackberries, boysenberries, gooseberries, mulberries

Beans: green beans, pole beans, snap beans, lima beans, fava beans, string beans

Cherries

Collards

Corn

Crookneck squash

Cucumbers

Figs

Grapefruit

Grapes

Mangoes

Melon: cantaloupe, watermelon

Nectarines

Okra

Parsnips

Papaya

Peaches

Pears

Peas: green peas, black-eyed peas

Peppers

Plumcots

Plums

Rhubarb

Summer squash

Swiss chard

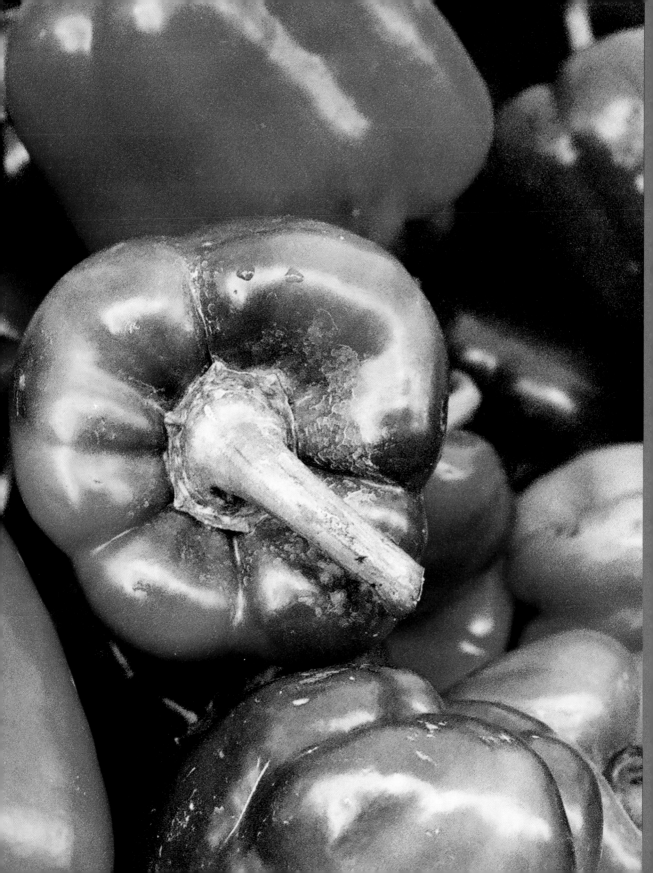

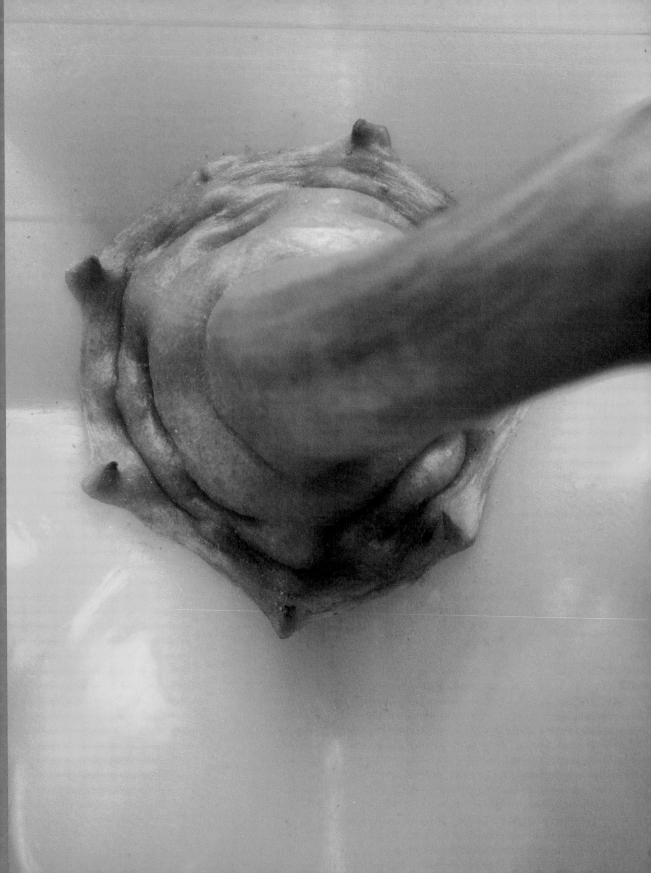

Tomato, Tarragon and Mostly Egg White Frittata

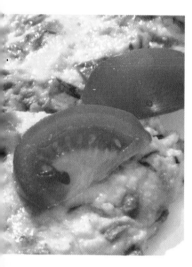

SERVES 8

8 large egg whites

2 large eggs

2 ounces parmesan, grated

1 tablespoon finely chopped fresh tarragon

½ teaspoon freshly ground black pepper

Pinch of sea salt

2 teaspoons butter

½ small onion, diced

6 organic plum tomatoes, seeded and diced

This recipe can be made with 12 egg whites and no yolks for an all egg white frittata.

1. Preheat oven to broil.

2. In a medium bowl, whisk eggs briefly until blended. Add half of the parmesan and all the tarragon, pepper, and salt.

3. Melt butter in a 9-or 10-inch nonstick, oven-safe sauté pan or skillet over medium-high heat. Add onion and sauté until soft. Add tomatoes and sauté for 2 to 3 minutes (or a little longer if they are very watery to allow water to evaporate). Pour egg mixture into pan and stir gently with a heat-resistant spatula. Cook for 4 to 5 minutes or until the egg mixture has set on the bottom and begins to set on top.

(continued)

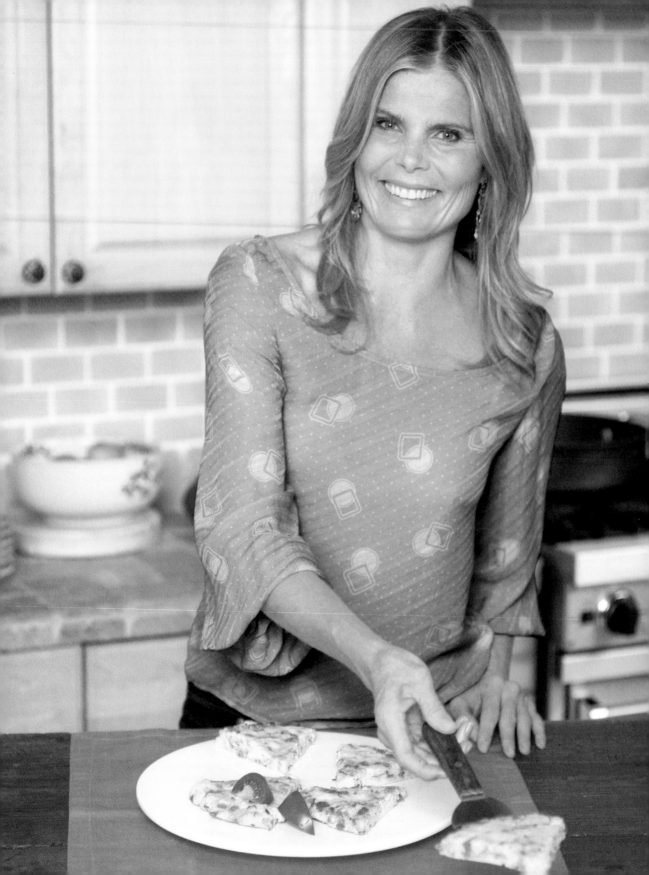

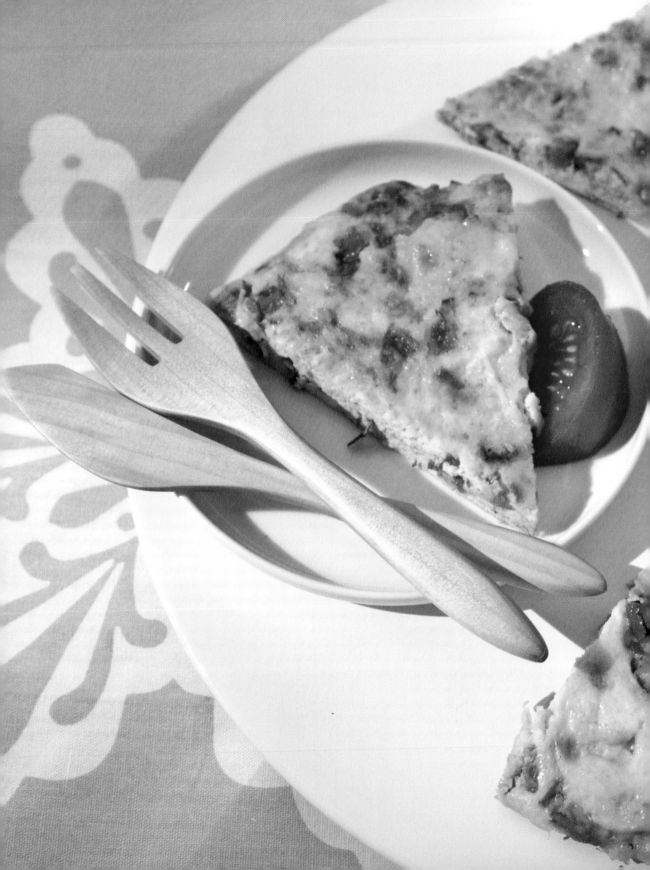

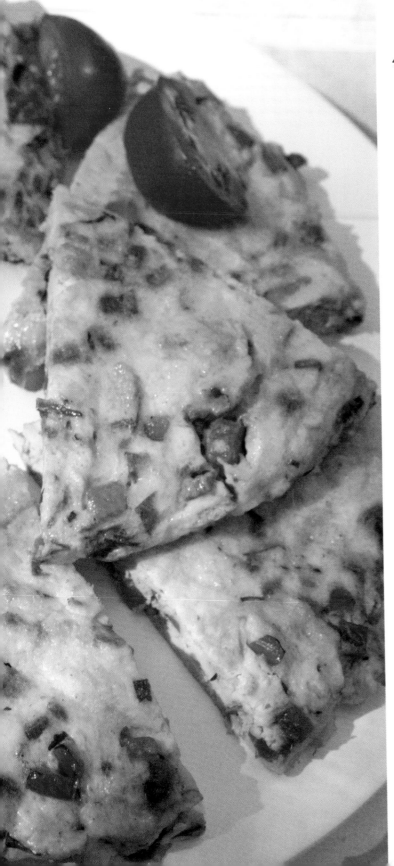

4. Sprinkle the remaining parmesan on top and place under broiler for 3 to 4 minutes until lightly browned and fluffy. Cool slightly, and then invert onto serving platter. Serve hot or at room temperature.

Cauliflower, Celery, and Green Pea Salad

Make this salad
when fresh peas
are available
for a healthy,
sweet crunch.
Use cleaned,
prepackaged
cauliflower
florets as a
time-saver.

SERVES 4–6

2   cups chopped cauliflower florets

1   cup diced celery

1   cup fresh or frozen and thawed shelled peas

¼   cup sliced green onions

1   cup Healthy Ranch Dressing (pg. 116)
    Lettuce leaves for serving, optional

1   cup coarsely chopped roasted cashews

1. Combine cauliflower, celery, peas, and green onions
   in a medium bowl. Cover and chill until ready to serve.

2. To serve, toss salad with Healthy Ranch Dressing, spoon
   on top of lettuce leaves, and sprinkle with cashews.

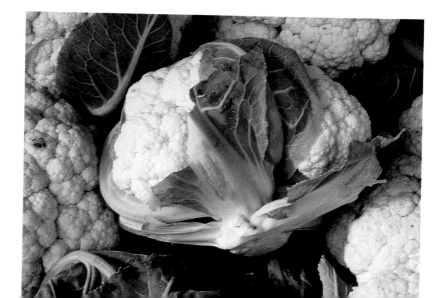

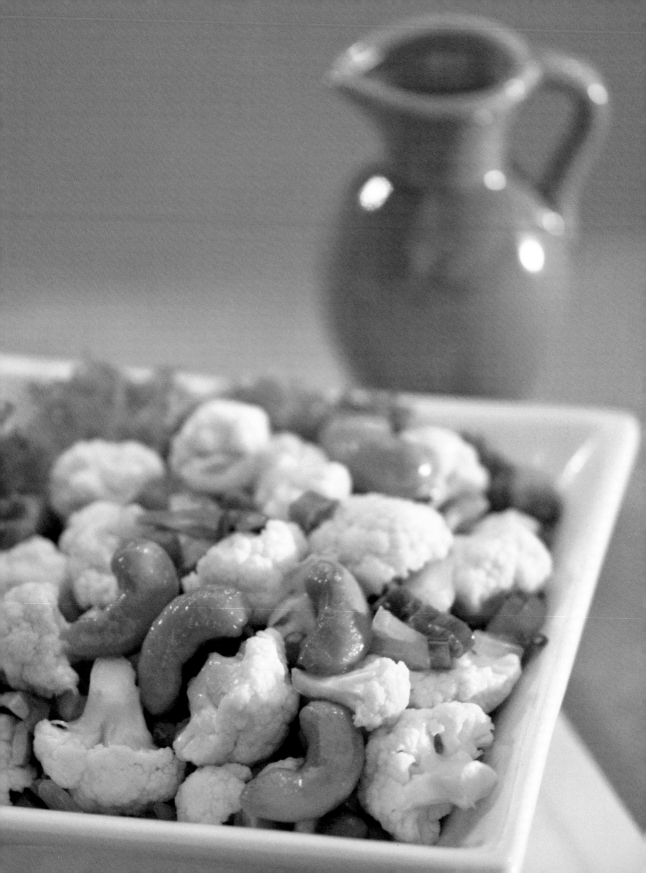

Healthy Ranch Dressing

MAKES 2 CUPS

Dressing
also makes a
wonderful dip
for crudités.

1 (6-ounce) package organic GMO-free silken tofu

2 tablespoons lemon juice

1 tablespoon olive oil

1 tablespoon chopped fresh parsley

2 cloves garlic, chopped

1 ½ tablespoons cider vinegar

Salt

Pepper

1. Place all ingredients in the work bowl of a food processor or blender. Blend until creamy and smooth. Refrigerate for up to 1 day.

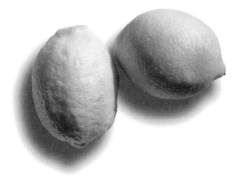

Raspberry Dressing

MAKES ABOUT 1 ¾ CUPS

- 1 cup organic raspberries
- ½ cup champagne vinegar
- 2 teaspoons Xylosweet
- 1 tablespoon Dijon mustard
  Pinch of sea salt
- ¼ cup almond oil

1. Place raspberries, vinegar, Xylosweet, mustard, and salt in a blender or food processor and process until well combined. Add oil slowly and process until creamy. Can be made 1 day ahead and stored, covered, in the refrigerator.

Substitute pomegranate vinegar for champagne vinegar. You can substitute frozen and thawed organic raspberries if fresh are unavailable.

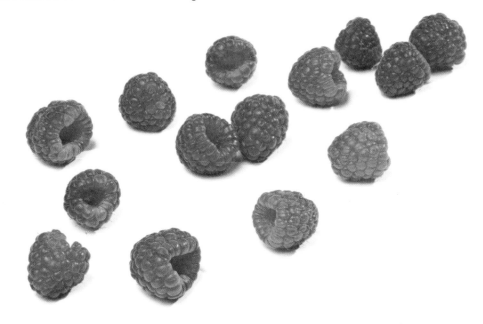

Watercress, Avocado, and Almond Salad

SERVES 4

For reduced fat, substitute 1 cup sliced water chestnuts for the avocado. Pomegranate seeds make a beautiful addition to this salad. Spinach or arugula can be substituted for the watercress.

1 bunch organic watercress, leaves and tender stems only

1 cup organic raspberries

1 ripe organic avocado, diced

½ cup whole toasted almonds

1 ¾ cups Raspberry Dressing (pg. 117)

I. Divide salad ingredients among four salad plates. Serve with Raspberry Dressing.

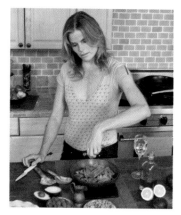
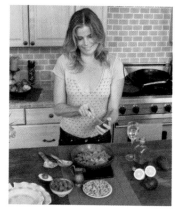
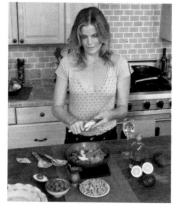

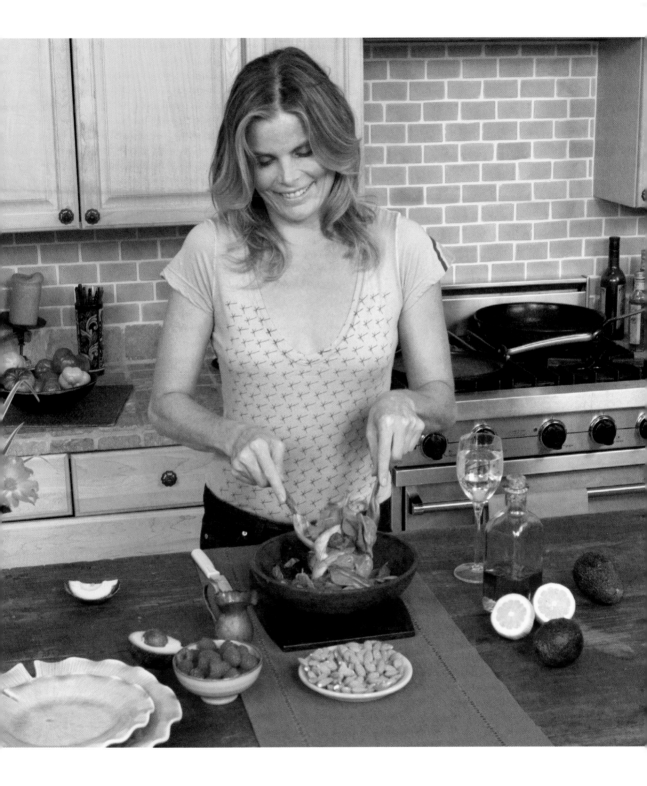

Vietnamese Chicken Lettuce Wraps with Mint-Basil Sauce

SERVES 4

Fish sauce, also known as *nam pla*, may be found in the Asian aisle of larger grocery stores. Used in moderation, it adds a nutty, almost cheesy flavor to dishes. For a vegan variation, replace the chicken with tempeh and the fish sauce with unseasoned rice vinegar.

Filling:

1 tablespoon coconut or olive oil

1 small onion, finely chopped

1 celery stalk, diced

2 garlic cloves, finely minced

1 tablespoon finely minced fresh ginger

1 pound ground organic chicken breast

1 (8-ounce) can water chestnuts, finely chopped

1 cup minced button mushrooms

2 tablespoons fish sauce

1 tablespoon tamari sauce, Bragg Liquid Aminos, or wheat-free soy sauce

1 teaspoon sesame oil

¼ teaspoon dried red pepper flakes

Mint-Basil Sauce:

⅓ cup tamari sauce, Bragg Liquid Aminos,
    or wheat-free soy sauce

⅓ cup unseasoned rice wine vinegar

2 teaspoons Asian garlic-chile paste or hot sauce

1 tablespoon fresh lime juice

2 teaspoons Xylosweet

2 tablespoons chopped fresh mint

2 tablespoons chopped fresh basil

16 butter lettuce or radicchio leaves

2 medium organic carrots, julienned or shredded

4 green onions, white and tender green parts only,
    thinly sliced

¼ cup coarsely chopped dry-roasted peanuts

1. To make the filling, heat coconut or olive oil in a large skillet over medium heat. Add onion and celery and sauté until soft, about 5 minutes. Add garlic and ginger and sauté until fragrant. Add ground chicken and sauté until cooked through and no longer pink, about 5 minutes, breaking up chicken as it cooks.

2. Add water chestnuts and mushrooms and sauté until mushrooms are cooked through, about 3 minutes. Add fish sauce, tamari sauce, sesame oil, and dried red pepper flakes. Mix well and remove from heat. Transfer to a large bowl and keep warm until you are ready to assemble wraps.

(continued)

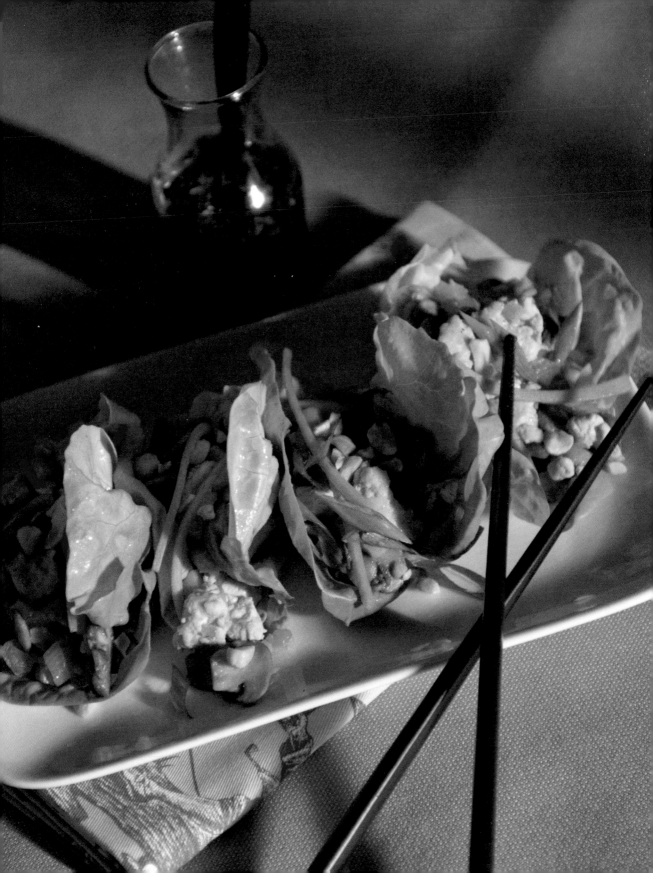

3. To make the sauce, combine all sauce ingredients in a small bowl and mix well.

4. To assemble the wraps, place lettuce leaves on a serving platter. Spoon about 2 tablespoons chicken mixture on top of each leaf. Top chicken with a few pieces of carrot and onion, a drizzle of sauce, and a sprinkle of peanuts. Serve immediately with remaining dipping sauce on the side.

Oven "Fried" Chicken

The coconut
oil adds flavor
to this recipe,
but you can use
butter if you
prefer.

SERVES 4

1   whole chicken, cut up

¾   cup brown rice flour

3   tablespoons paprika

3   tablespoons garlic powder

1   tablespoon sea salt

2   teaspoons freshly ground black pepper

6   tablespoons coconut oil

1. Preheat oven to 375°F.

2. Pat chicken pieces dry with paper towels.

3. Combine flour, paprika, garlic powder, salt, and pepper on
   a plate or pie pan. Set aside.

4. Rub chicken pieces in coconut oil to saturate all sides,
   and then press into flour mixture to coat. Shake off
   excess and place chicken pieces in a large baking dish.

5. Bake for 30 to 40 minutes or until the chicken is cooked
   through completely and the juices run clear.

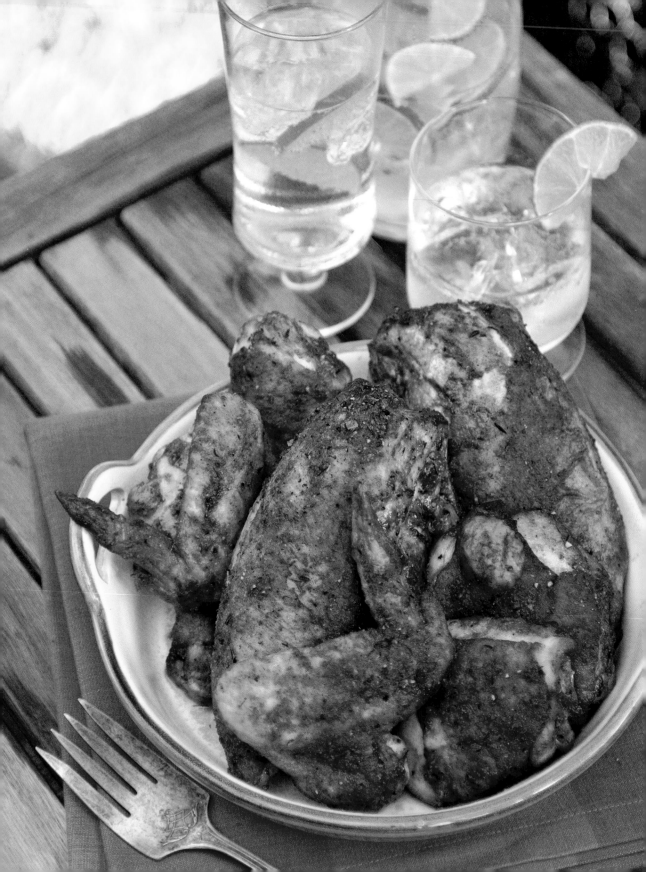

Grilled Scallops with Fennel and Peppers

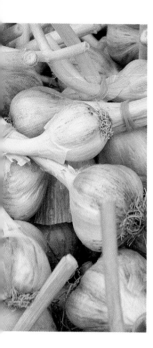

SERVES 4

2 tablespoons coconut or olive oil

1 tablespoon unsalted butter

1 large organic fennel bulb, trimmed and julienned, reserving fronds for garnish

1 large organic red bell pepper, stem and seeds removed, julienned

1 large organic yellow or orange bell pepper, stem and seeds removed, julienned

2 teaspoons Xylosweet

1 garlic clove, minced
   Sea salt
   Freshly ground black pepper

8 large sea scallops, muscle removed if necessary (about 12 ounces)

1. Heat 1 tablespoon of the oil and all the butter over medium-low heat in a large sauté pan. Add fennel, peppers, and Xylosweet and sauté, stirring frequently, until fennel caramelizes, 10 to 12 minutes. Add garlic, salt, and pepper and sauté until garlic becomes fragrant, 2 to 3 minutes. Remove from heat and cover to keep warm.

2. Preheat grill pan over high heat.

3. Pat scallops dry with paper towels and brush both sides with oil. Season with salt and pepper. Grill scallops until they have developed deep golden grill marks on both sides and are opaque throughout, being careful not to overcook.

4. To serve, spoon warm fennel mixture onto individual dinner plates. Top with grilled scallops. Garnish with reserved fresh fennel fronds.

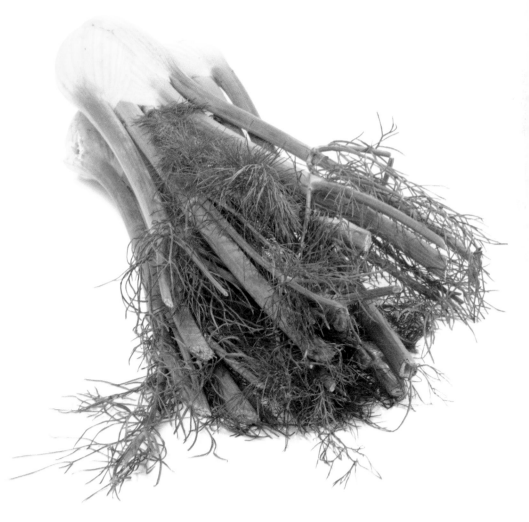

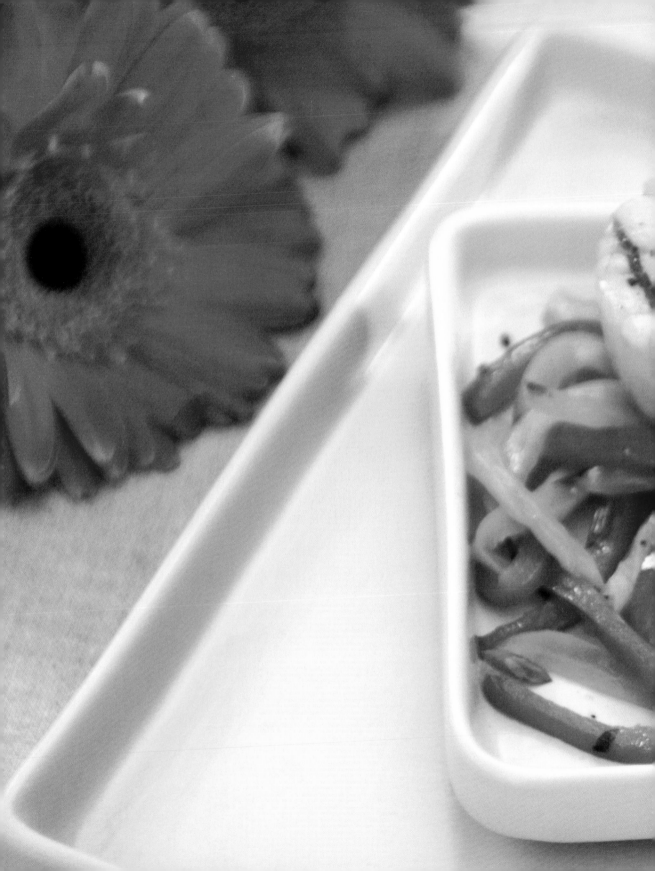

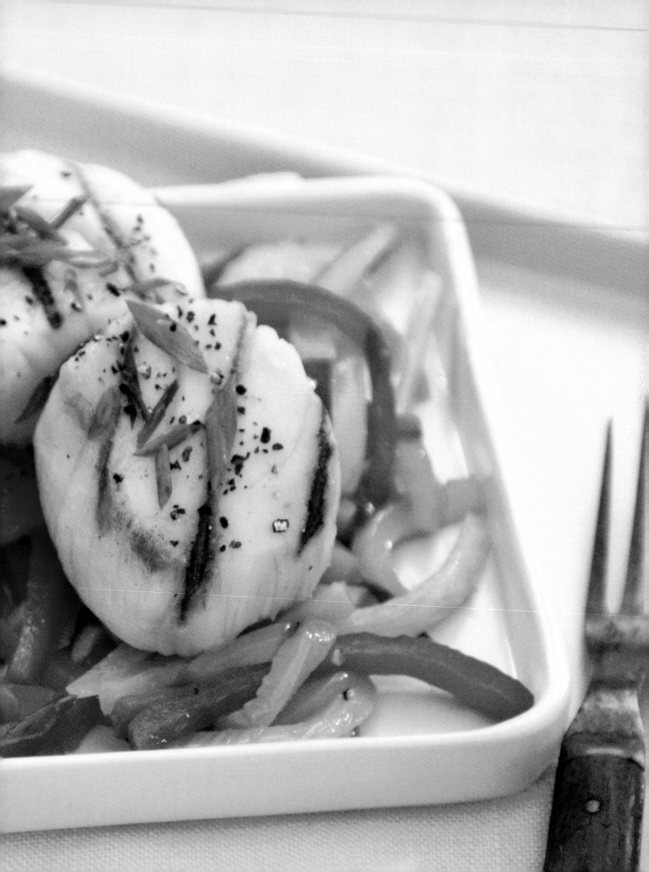

Summer Squash "Linguini" with Chicken, Goat Cheese, and Basil

SERVES 4

For a vegetarian variation to this recipe, replace the chicken with firm tofu.

2   tablespoons coconut or olive oil

2   (4-ounce) boneless, skinless chicken breasts, preferably free-range organic, cut into ½-inch pieces

Sea salt

Freshly ground black pepper

1   tablespoon unsalted butter

1   tablespoon minced shallot

1   garlic clove, minced

¼   cup chicken broth, vegetable broth, or water

3   small organic green zucchini, julienned

3   small organic yellow zucchini, julienned

¼   cup julienned fresh basil

5   ounces goat cheese, crumbled

1. Heat oil in a large sauté pan over medium heat. Season chicken pieces with salt and pepper and sauté until the outside is golden and the chicken is cooked through and no longer pink. Remove from pan with a slotted spoon into a bowl, cover to keep warm and set aside. Drain all but 1 tablespoon of oil from pan.

2. Add butter to pan. Add shallot and sauté until it becomes soft, about 3 to 4 minutes. Add garlic and sauté until fragrant. Add chicken broth, vegetable broth, or water; then add zucchini and sauté for about 3 to 4 minutes or just until soft. Remove from heat. Add chicken and basil, season with salt and pepper, and stir to combine. Divide among four individual dinner plates and top with the crumbled goat cheese. Serve immediately.

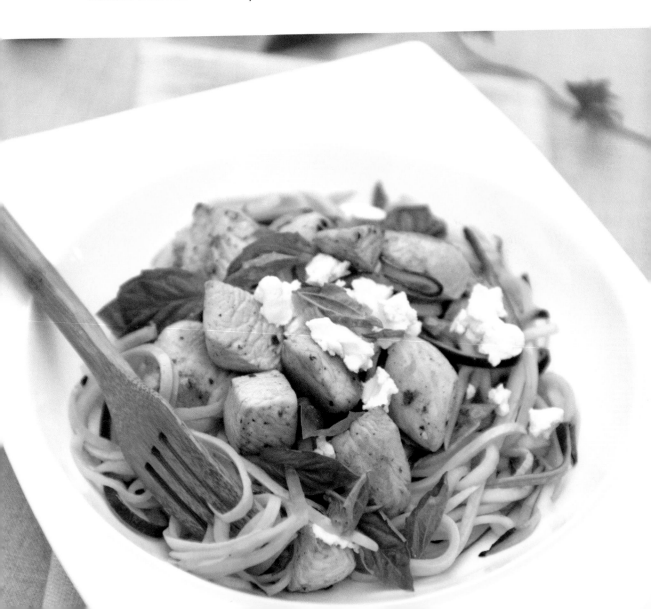

Farmers' Market Heirloom Gazpacho

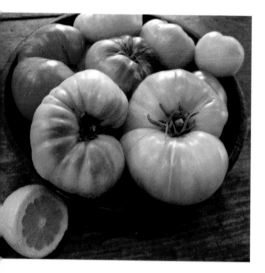

SERVES 8

6 large, ripe, red and yellow organic heirloom tomatoes, diced

1 small red onion, diced

2 stalks organic celery, diced

1 organic seedless cucumber, diced

1 organic red bell pepper, stem and seeds removed, diced

1 small jalapeño pepper, stem, seeds, and veins removed, minced

3 garlic cloves, minced

¼ cup chopped fresh parsley

¼ cup chopped fresh basil

2 tablespoons chopped fresh chives

¼ cup sherry vinegar

¼ cup olive oil

2 tablespoons fresh lemon juice

2 teaspoons Xylosweet

4 cups organic, low-sodium tomato juice

Sea salt

Freshly ground black pepper

1. Combine all ingredients in a large, nonreactive mixing bowl. Place half the mixture in the bowl of a food processor or blender and puree until smooth. Return pureed mixture to mixing bowl and stir to combine. Cover bowl tightly and refrigerate 4 to 8 hours to allow flavors to blend. Serve cold in soup bowls.

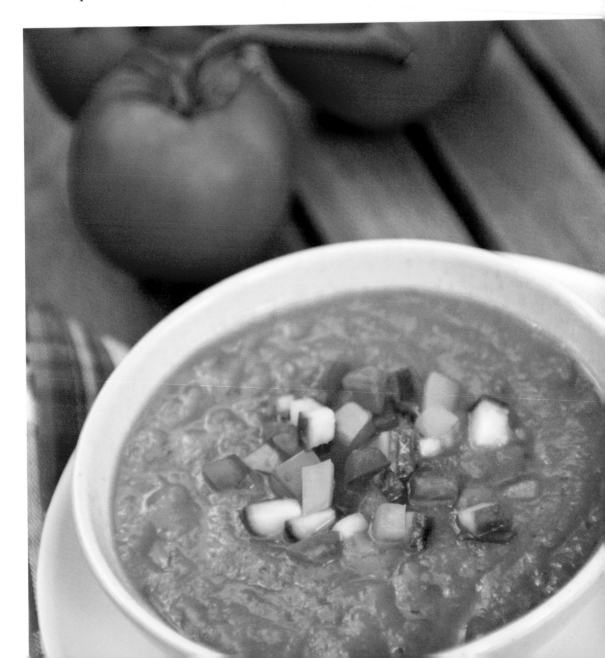

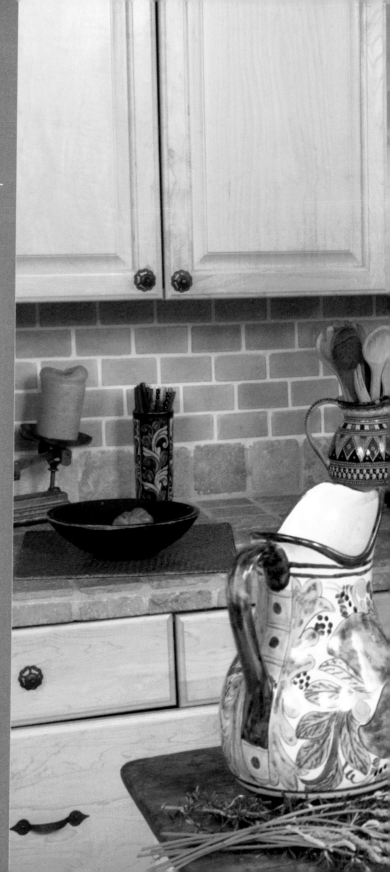

You don't have to be an expert in the kitchen to make great food. As long as you have a little bit of familiarity with different ingredients, oils, and fresh herbs, you can create like an artist, and put an explosion of colors together into a rainbow on your plate. Making a meal becomes like dipping a paintbrush into the palette and playing, always wondering what that canvas is going to look like when it's ready.

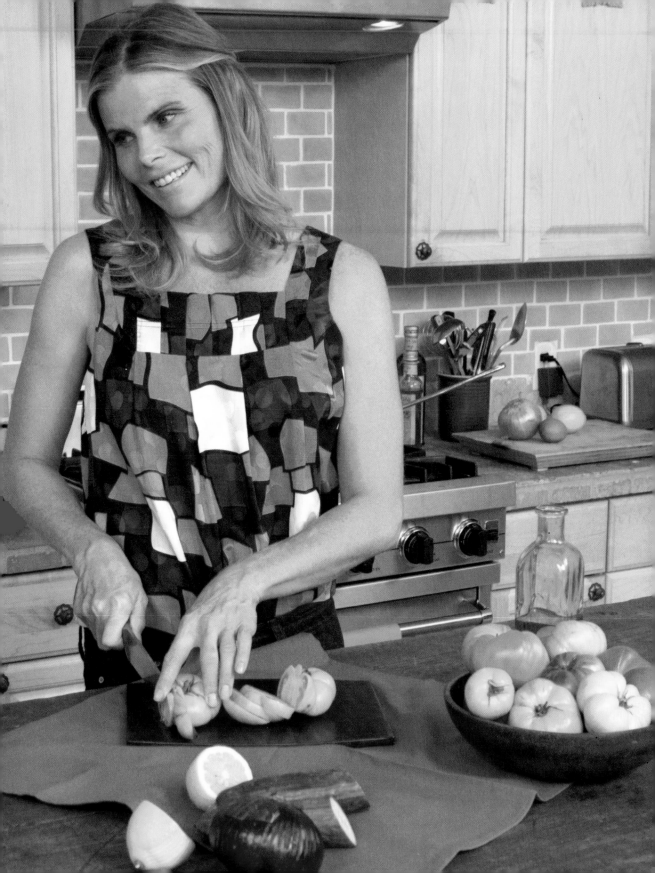

Pesto Halibut with Braised Fennel

If halibut is
unavailable,
you can
substitute
scrod, cod,
snapper,
or sea bass.

SERVES 4

2   tablespoons unsalted butter

2   large fennel bulbs, trimmed, quartered

2   garlic cloves, whole, peeled and smashed

¼   teaspoon dried red pepper flakes

   Organic vegetable broth

   Sea salt

   Freshly ground black pepper

1   tablespoon coconut or olive oil

4   (4- to 6-ounce) halibut fillets, skin removed

8   ounces fresh organic basil pesto sauce
    (purchased or homemade)

1. Melt 1 tablespoon of the butter over medium heat in a heavy skillet large enough to hold fennel in a single layer. Add fennel, garlic, and red pepper flakes and enough broth to just cover the fennel. Bring liquid to a boil, reduce heat, cover and simmer until fennel is very tender, about 20 minutes. Remove from heat and stir in the remaining 1 tablespoon butter. Season with salt and pepper if desired. Cover to keep warm.

2. Preheat oven to 350°F.

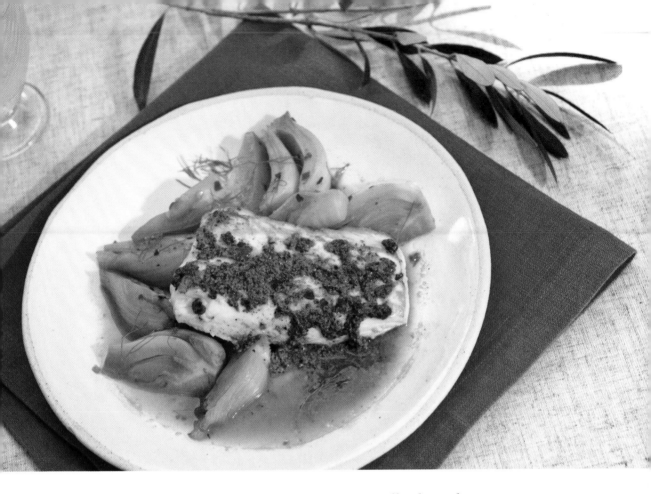

3. Pat fillets dry with paper towels and season on all sides with
   salt and pepper. Heat oil in a large, heavy oven-proof skillet
   over medium heat. Add fillets and sear on each side until golden,
   about 2 minutes per side. Remove from heat. Top each fillet
   with about 2 tablespoons pesto sauce and place skillet in oven
   until fish is cooked through and flaky, about 5 minutes.

4. To serve, place fennel along with a little broth in shallow
   bowls. Place a halibut fillet on top, and serve extra pesto sauce
   on the side.

Portobello Mushrooms with Spinach and Goat Cheese

SERVES 4

Filling can be used for stuffing small mushrooms as well. Decrease baking time accordingly. This recipe serves twice as many when served as a first course rather than an entrée.

2 tablespoons coconut or olive oil

4 large portobello mushrooms, stem and gills removed

  Sea salt

  Freshly ground black pepper

1 small onion, diced

2 garlic cloves, minced

1 (10-ounce) package frozen spinach, thawed and drained

2 tablespoons finely chopped fresh parsley

2 teaspoons finely chopped fresh thyme

¼ teaspoon dried red pepper flakes

3 ounces soft goat cheese, crumbled (¼ cup)

4 tablespoons grated parmesan

1. Preheat oven to 350°F. Brush mushrooms with 1 tablespoon of the oil and season with salt and pepper. Place on a baking sheet covered with parchment paper or aluminum foil and set aside.

2. Heat the remaining 1 tablespoon oil in a large sauté pan over medium heat. Add onion and sauté until softened. Add garlic and sauté until fragrant. Add spinach and sauté just until all

liquid has evaporated. Add herbs and red pepper flakes, and season with salt and pepper to taste. Remove from heat. Gently stir in goat cheese until combined.

3. Divide filling among mushrooms and stuff generously. Sprinkle with parmesan and a few red pepper flakes. Bake until mushrooms soften and filling is bubbling, about 20 minutes. Serve immediately.

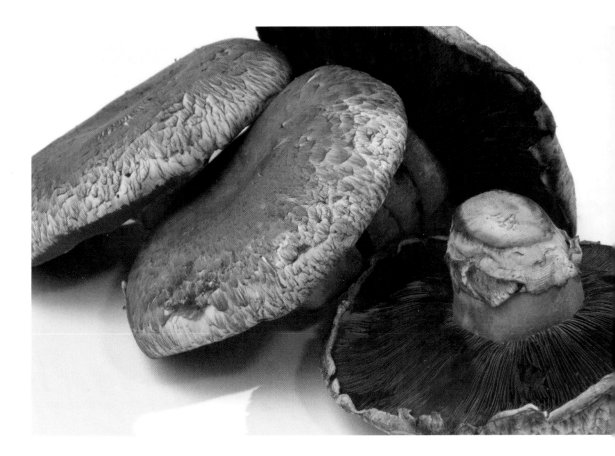

Fresh Raspberry Soufflé

MAKES 6 (4-OUNCE) SOUFFLÉS

This elegant dessert can also be made in one large soufflé pan. Increase oven time to about 25 minutes or until soufflé has puffed and top is golden.

Unsalted butter for preparing ramekins

⅔ cup plus 3 tablespoons Xylosweet, plus extra for preparing ramekins

4 cups fresh organic raspberries, reserving 12 berries for garnish

1 teaspoon fresh organic lemon zest

2 tablespoons organic brown rice flour

6 large egg whites, room temperature

1. Preheat oven to 375°F. Butter 6 individual 4-ounce ramekins. Coat with a little Xylosweet and shake out any excess.

2. Purée raspberries with 3 tablespoons Xylosweet in a food processor or blender. Strain with a fine mesh strainer into a heavy medium saucepan, pressing on solids. Add flour and whisk to blend. Continue whisking over medium heat until mixture boils and thickens to consistency of a very thick pudding, about 3 minutes. Transfer mixture to large mixing bowl and cool completely at room temperature.

(continued)

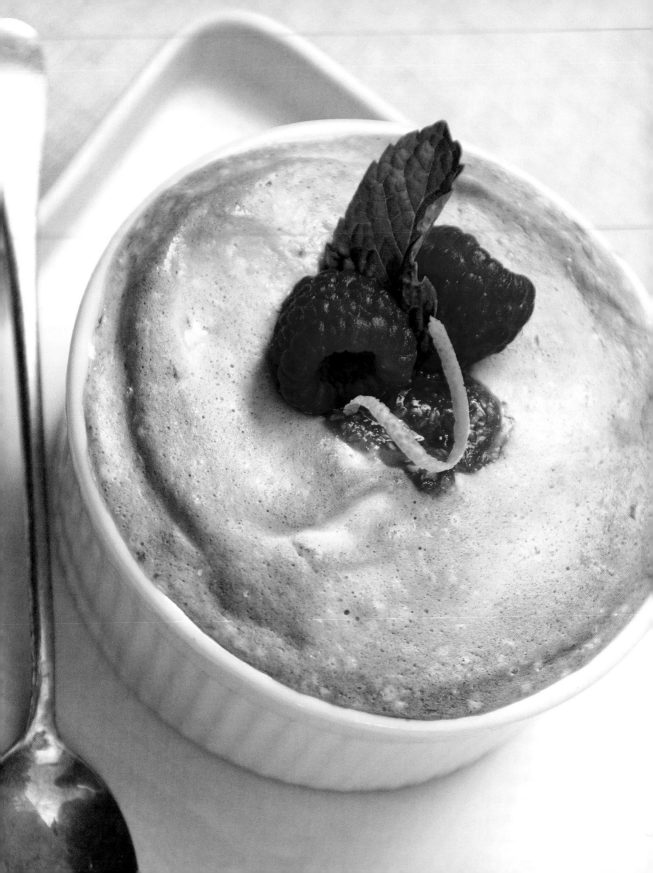

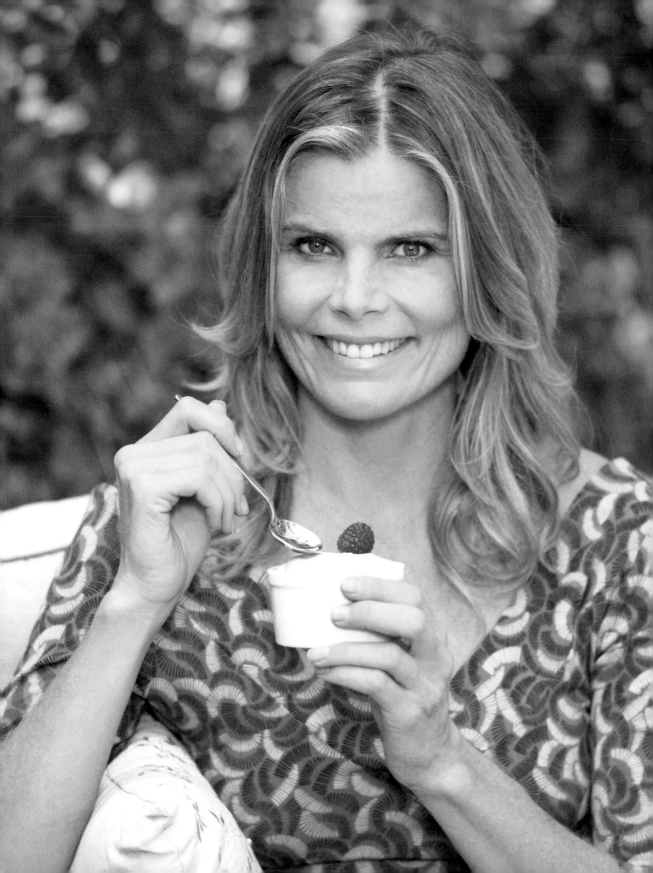

3. Whisk egg whites to soft peaks in another large mixing bowl. Gradually add the remaining ⅔ cup Xylosweet while whisking to stiff peaks. Whisk by hand one-third of whites into raspberry mixture to lighten, then fold in the remaining whites and lemon zest being careful not to overmix and deflate the whites too much. Divide mixture among prepared ramekins. Bake until puffed and golden on top, about 15 to 18 minutes. Serve immediately (soufflés will fall as they cool).

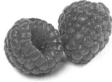

Broiled Peaches with Blackberry Puree

SERVES 4

2 pints fresh organic blackberries

2 tablespoons plus ½ teaspoon Xylosweet

2 tablespoons fresh, organic lemon juice

2 large fresh ripe organic peaches, halved, pits removed

1. Preheat broiler on high.

2. Puree blackberries with 2 tablespoons of the Xylosweet and 1 tablespoon of the lemon juice in a food processor or blender. Strain through a fine mesh strainer into a small mixing bowl pushing on solids to extract all of the pulp. Set aside.

3. Place peach halves on a baking sheet covered with parchment paper or aluminum foil. Sprinkle with the remaining lemon juice and Xylosweet. Place under broiler and cook until the tops of peaches begin to brown, about 3 minutes. Remove from oven to cool slightly.

4. To serve, place a couple of spoonfuls of puree in individual shallow serving bowls or dessert plates. Top each with a peach half. Serve additional puree on the side.

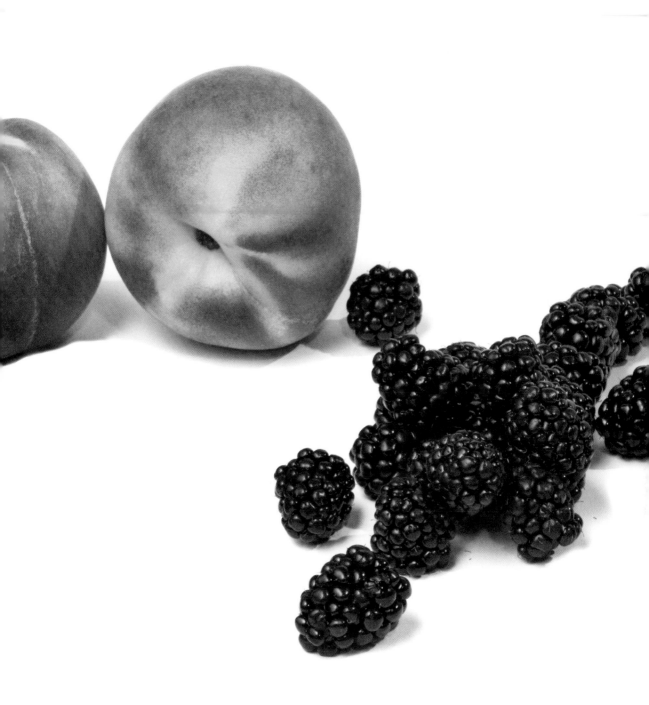

Lemon Custard

Garnish with
lemon wedges or
serve with fresh
organic berries.

½ cup Xylosweet

4 large eggs, at room temperature

Pinch of sea salt

1 ¾ cups low-fat milk

1 organic lemon, zested and juiced

1. In medium bowl, whisk together Xylosweet, eggs, and salt.
Set aside.

2. In large saucepan, heat milk over medium heat until tiny
bubbles appear around edges of pan. Remove from heat.

3. Slowly add hot milk to egg mixture, ¼ cup at a time,
stirring constantly to gently heat the eggs without cooking
them. Pour mixture back into saucepan.

4. Cook over medium-low heat, stirring constantly,
until mixture has thickened and coats the back of
a spoon. Do not allow to boil or mixture will curdle.
Remove from heat.

5. Strain through a fine mesh strainer into another bowl.
Stir in lemon zest and juice.

6. Nest bowl with hot custard into a larger bowl which has been partially filled with ice water. Let custard sit, stirring frequently, until it has cooled completely.

7. Pour custard into individual dessert cups and serve, or cover tightly with plastic wrap and refrigerate for up to a day.

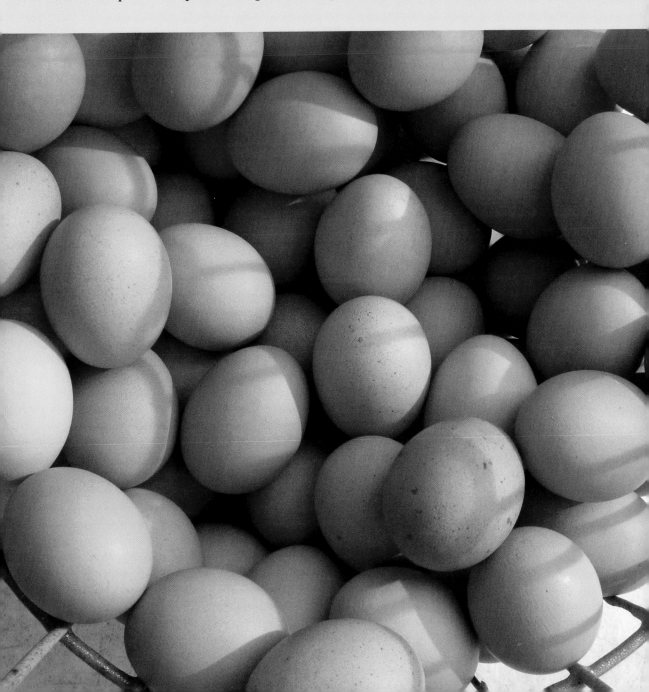

Mariel's Peach Slush

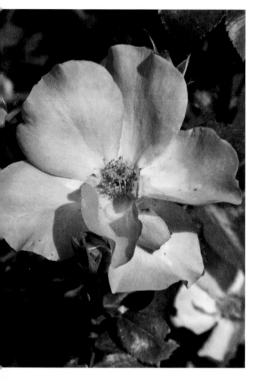

SERVES 2

2 peaches, pitted

⅔ cup cut seedless watermelon

1 cup ice cubes

1 scoop (about 2 tablespoons) whey protein isolate powder

2 cups sparkling water

Mint sprigs for garnish

1. Place peaches, watermelon, ice cubes, and protein powder in a blender and puree until smooth. Add sparkling water and pulse to combine. Pour into two glasses, garnish with mint sprigs, and enjoy!

For flavor, fiber, and loads of vitamin C, blend in a few mint leaves or a quarter cup of raspberries.

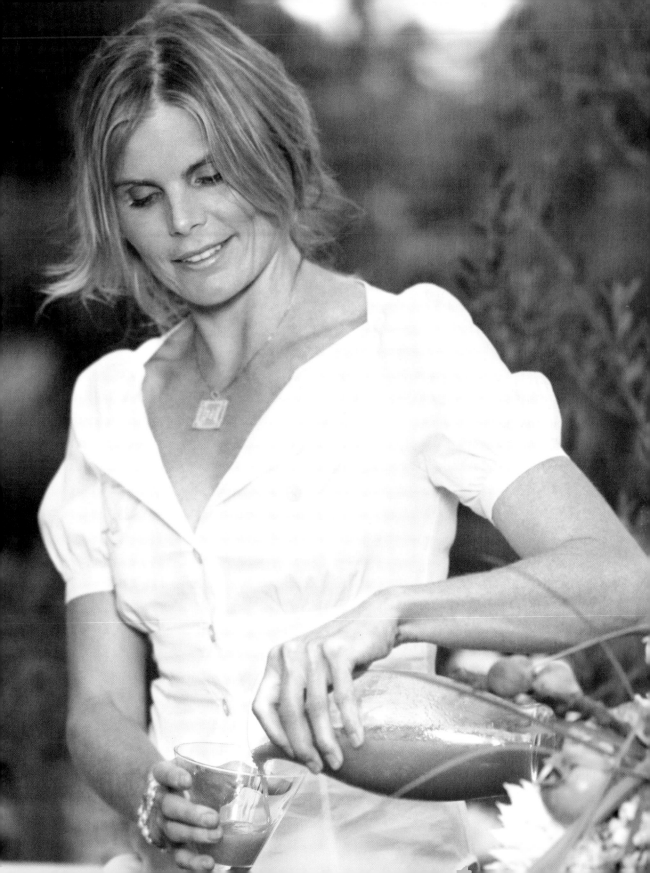

Simple and Satisfying Entertainment

Summertime invites us to share our table and experience the joy of eating communally. Sultry evenings let us drop fears about perfection and ease into cooking for a crowd without stress or worry. After years of serving up food for family, friends, and sometimes casts and crews, I have my system down.

1 Spend an hour doing morning prep work: **Setting the table and doing prep work in the morning, or even** the evening before people come, is a little time-management trick that makes entertaining seem doable. Cut any veggies that need dicing or slicing for your recipes and refrigerate them. A spray of lemon juice keeps their color and flavor intact.

2 Don't fret over a formal dinner setting: **Summer tables are about festivity. Choose colored recycled napkins** and stick the utensils in colorful glasses. Put knives and forks in a bright yellow mug, your spoons in cobalt blue, and your table looks like a party.

3 Serve interesting, nonalcoholic drinks in place of sodas: **Coconut water is a perfect, refreshing drink** for hot weather. It is very hydrating, full of electrolytes, but free of the chemicals or excessive sugars of a sports drink, and it tastes fabulous. Mix with mint for an extra kick. Brewing some aromatic teas and then icing them in a pitcher with fresh herbs or fruit works well too. Delegate your friends to bring some drinks, but stipulate, "No sodas!"

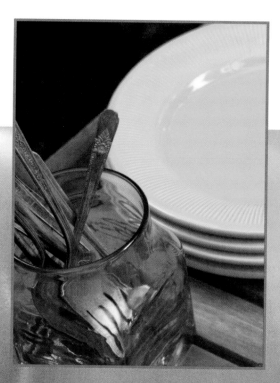

4 Plant some snacks around the kitchen: **Have some munchies ready for your guests like Spicy Mixed Nuts, Savory Cheese Blisscuits, and Pumpkin Walnut Balls, because summer equals late arrivals and the early birds get hungry. Crudités can be bought precut and served with any of my dressings.**

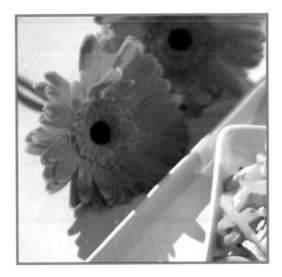

5 Make pick 'n' mix serving plates: **Divide the components of the meal amongst serving plates and bowls of different shapes and sizes. Protein on one tray; salad in another bowl; dressing, nuts, and other sides in their own dishes. Look at it as a whole picture and make it pretty. A few flowers can decorate the platters. Let guests compile a plate that appeals to their senses.**

6 Add an old-fashioned element: **For a super simple but fun dessert, pass around a soda fountain-style whipped cream dispenser, and let guests squirt their own organic cream over fresh summer berries.**

7 Don't rush: **Eating in summer means there's no sense of time. People drift in when the cooking has begun and hang out by the stove or barbecue. The joy is that the preparation, cooking, and socializing are one and the same. You eat when the food is ready and even still, it can sit for latecomers! Piping hot isn't so important in August. Let it all be as it is. Everything about this season is casual.**

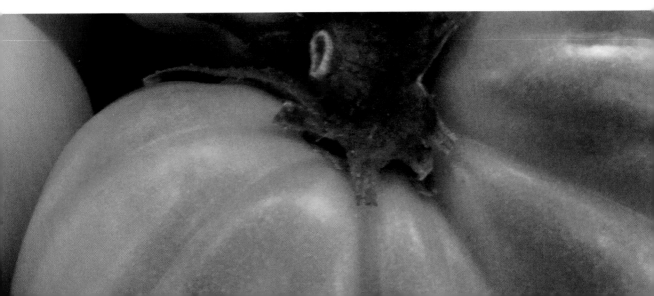

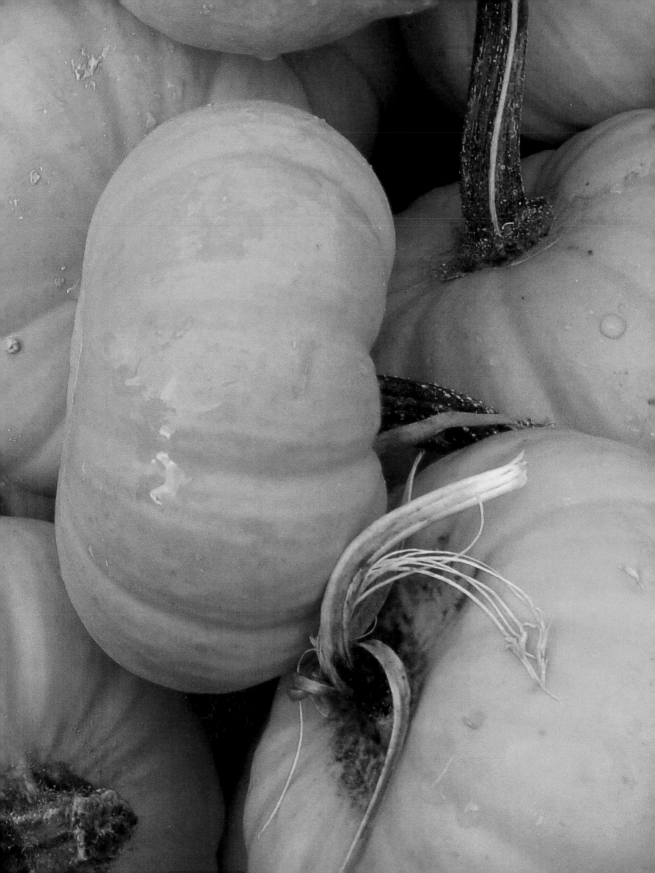

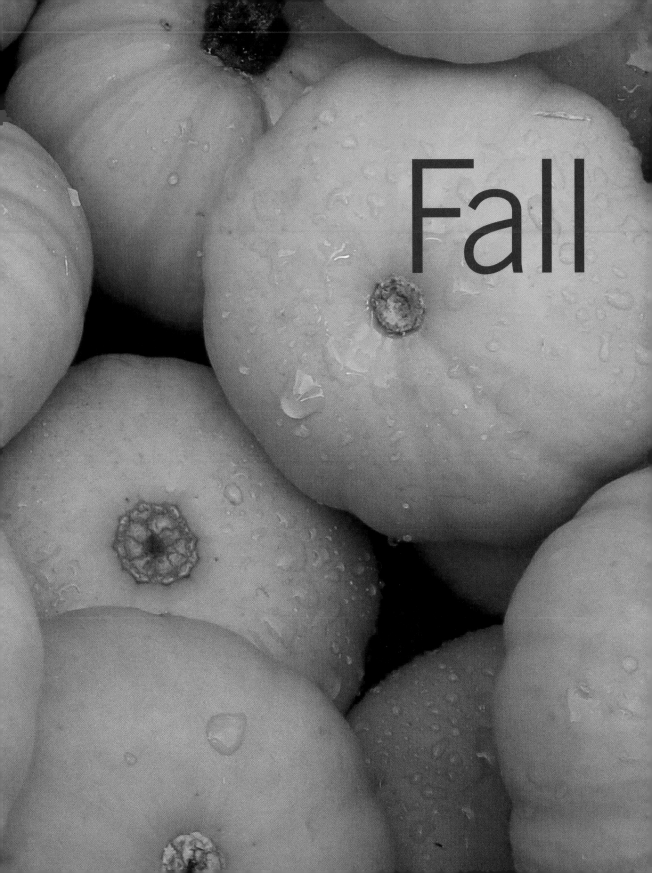

Fall

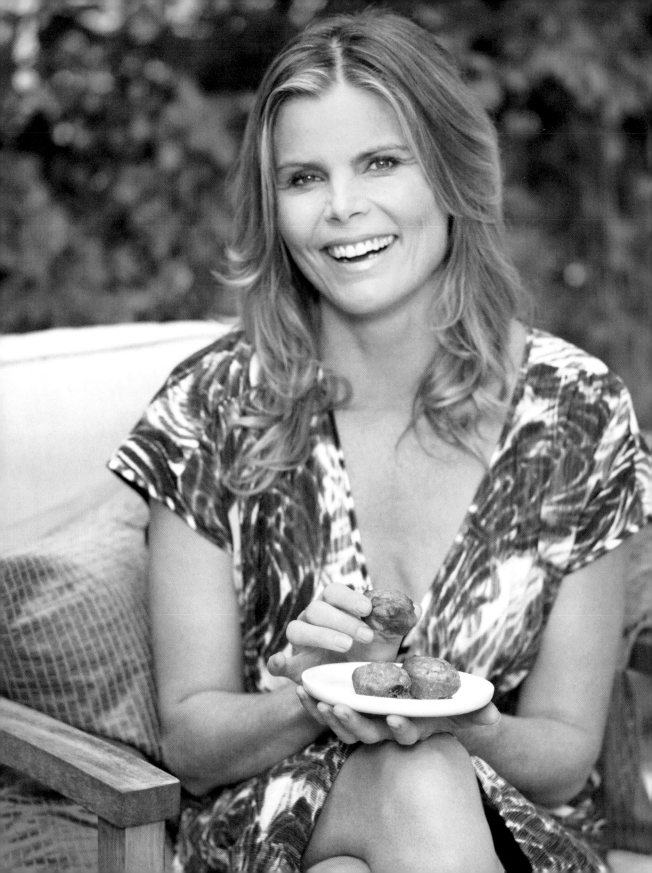

Eating off the Land

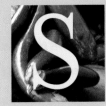

Some of my favorite food memories are set in the fall. In the mountains where I grew up, the August heat bakes you one day; the next there's a chill in the air announcing the start of bundled-up responsibility: Get up for school, pull on woolly socks, and stick Chapstick in your pocket! Even the earth seems more serious as it prepares to be silenced by blankets of snow. The chill brings a new set of smells and sensations. The aroma of sage fills your nose, your body feels denser, and your breath is deeper. And most of all there's a clean, fierce hunger. All the busyness sparks a fire in the belly and, like the stove inside your house, the body asks for some real fuel.

that only needs a quick grill or sauté. Because it's made of fermented soy, it avoids the health dangers of unfermented soy milks, tofu, and processed vegetarian meals that are now such a part of the Western diet. Soy in Asian countries is a condiment, not intended to be a major protein source. I feel it is a food to be consumed in moderation.

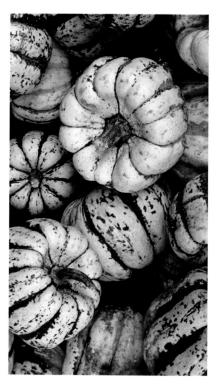

When we make a shift around Thanksgiving, it signals a year-round commitment to eating well that is bigger than counting calories. If special events no longer trigger a run on store-bought treats, you know you've cracked it: you've made simple, whole foods a part of your ritual. When you put seasonal, sustainable foods together, using as much organic as possible, automatically making good choices about the quality of the ingredients, it is, for lack of a

Fall is about earthy colors and flavors.

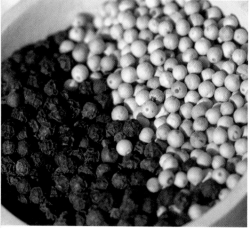

better term, an act of self-love. You're not just cooking: you're truly caring for yourself, for your family, and loved ones.

Fall Produce

Almonds	Green beans
Apples	Kiwis
Asian pears	Melon
Beans	Parsnips
Beets	Pears
Blueberries	Pumpkins
Broccoli	Persimmons
Brussels sprouts	Rapini
Cabbage	Sunchokes
Cauliflower	Sweet potatoes
Chestnuts	Swiss chard
Endive	Tangerines
Fennel	Turnips
Grapefruit	Yams

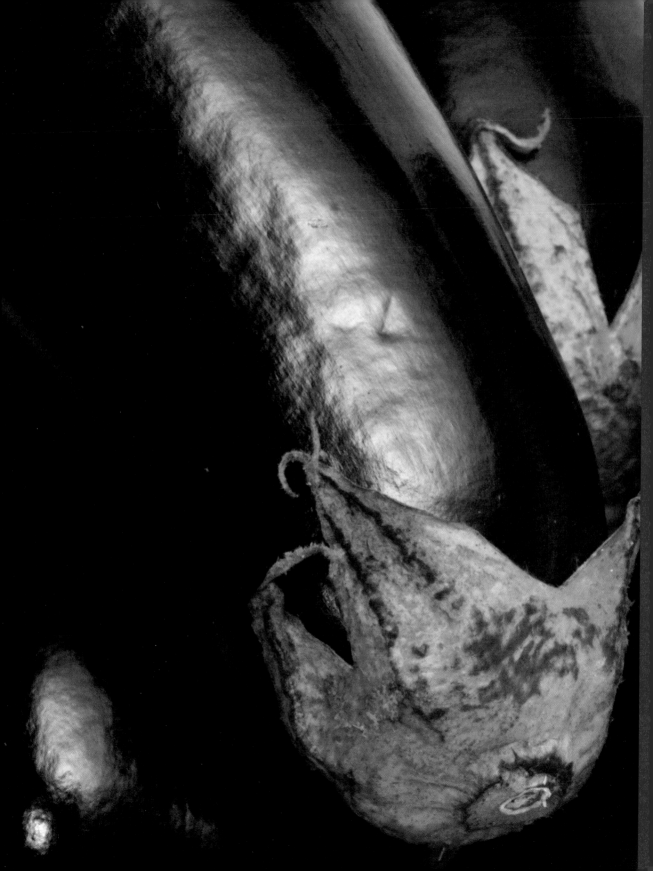

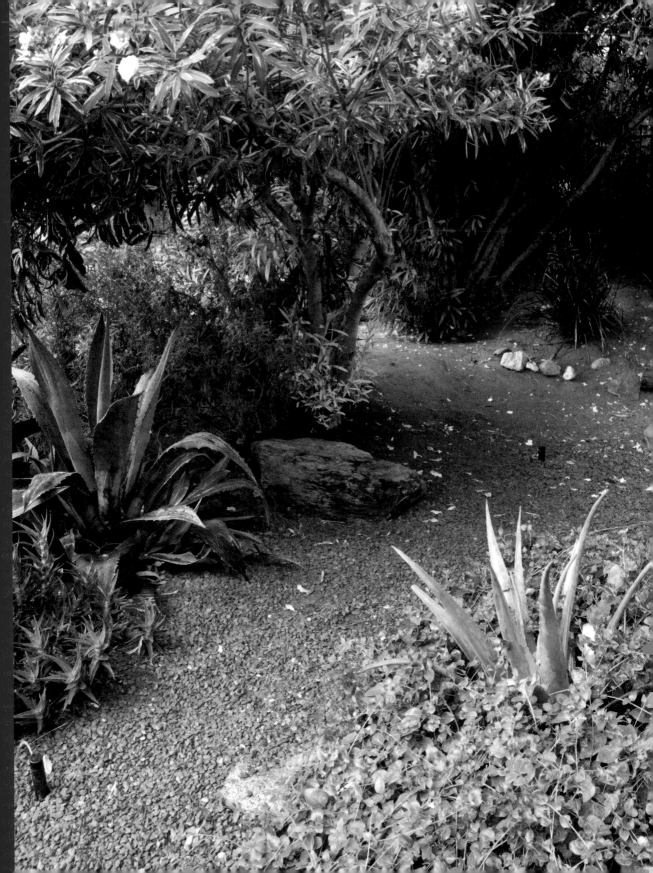

Poached Eggs on Wilted Greens

SERVES 6

- 1 teaspoon white wine vinegar
- 12 large eggs
- 3 tablespoons water
- 2 heads escarole, or 2 bunches Swiss chard or baby spinach, coarsely chopped
- 1 teaspoon salt
- ½ teaspoon pepper
- 2 plum tomatoes, cut into small wedges or diced

1. Fill a pot with 2 inches of water. Add vinegar and bring to a light simmer over medium heat

2. Begin gently cracking the eggs, one at a time, closely into the pot (do these in batches of three to be sure not to overcrowd the pot).

3. Once the whites begin to set up, but the yolks are still soft and runny, carefully remove each egg with a slotted spoon and set aside in a warm area.

(continued)

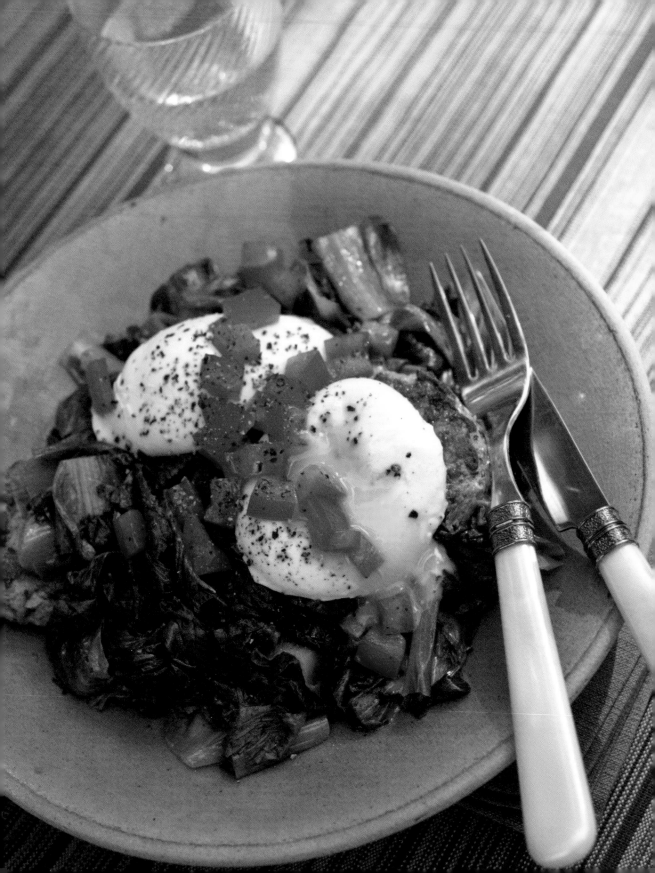

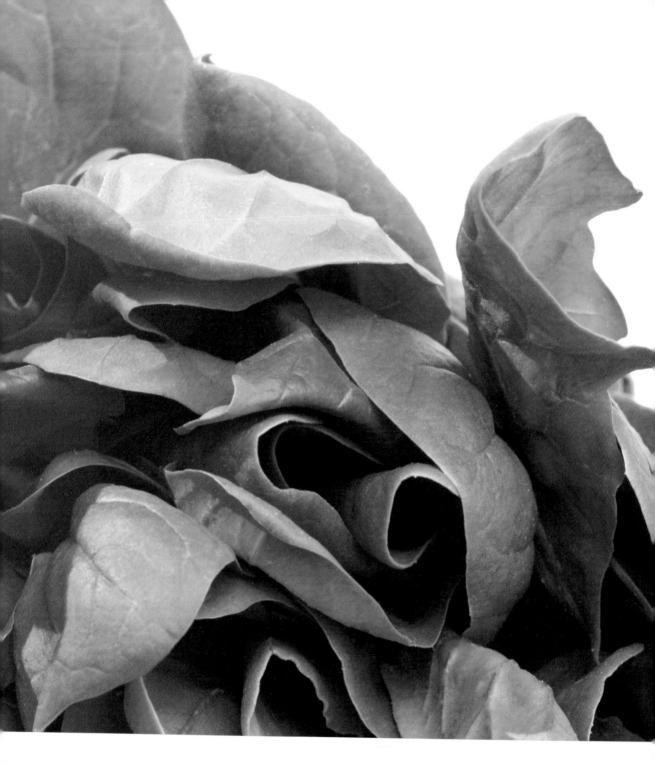

4. Place 3 tablespoons of water in a large sauté pan with the greens. Heat until barely wilted (the warm eggs will wilt the greens more).

5. Season greens with salt and pepper, drain slightly to remove excess liquid, and divide the greens onto 6 individual plates. Place tomato wedges around the plate or sprinkle the diced tomatoes on top.

6. Top each plate with 2 poached eggs and serve.

7. As an option add Turkey and Veggie Sausages (pg. 42).

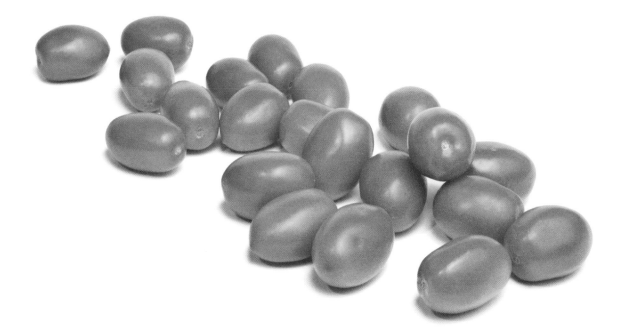

Cranberry Blisscuit Mini Muffins

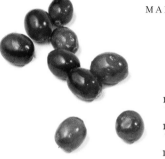

MAKES 12 MINI MUFFINS

Coconut oil for greasing muffin tin

1 cup almond meal

½ cup plus 1 tablespoon whey protein isolate powder

½ cup Xylosweet

¼ cup finely shredded unsweetened coconut

3 tablespoons coconut flour

1 teaspoon baking powder

1 teaspoon xanthan gum

½ cup coconut oil

1 large egg

2 large egg whites

¾ teaspoon vanilla extract

½ teaspoon almond extract

1 cup fat-free milk

2 ounces organic goat cheese

⅓ cup dried cranberries

1. Preheat oven to 300°F. Lightly grease a mini muffin tin with coconut oil.

2. Place almond meal, whey powder, Xylosweet, shredded coconut, coconut flour, baking powder, and xanthan gum in a large bowl and mix together well.

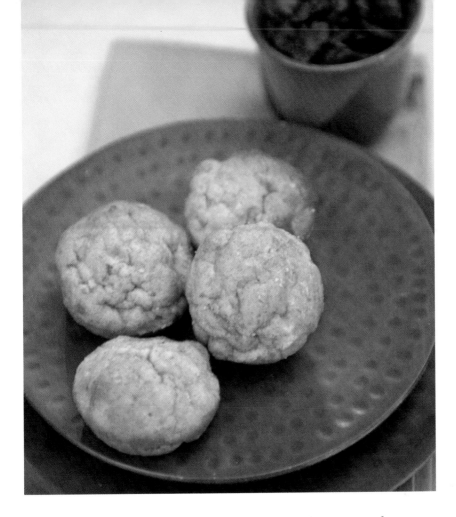

3. In a medium bowl whisk together coconut oil, egg, egg whites, vanilla and almond extracts, milk, and goat cheese. Pour into dry ingredients and mix together well. Stir in cranberries.

4. Spoon mixture into prepared muffin tin, filling compartments to the top, and bake for 25 to 30 minutes until cooked through.

5. Let cool before storing in an airtight container for up to 3 days. Or freeze for up to 1 month.

Sliced Grilled Tempeh in Wild Mushroom Sauce with Peppers

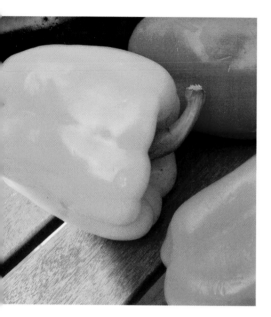

SERVES 4

2 tablespoons coconut or olive oil

1 small onion, diced

2 garlic cloves, minced

1 large organic red bell pepper, diced

1 large organic orange or yellow bell pepper, diced

8 ounces fresh wild mushrooms

2 cups vegetable broth

Sea salt

Freshly ground black pepper

2 (8-ounce) packages tempeh

1. Heat 1 tablespoon of the oil over medium heat in a large sauté pan. Add onion and sauté until softened, about 5 minutes. Add garlic and sauté just until fragrant. Add peppers and mushrooms and sauté another 2 to 3 minutes.

2. Add broth and bring to a boil; then reduce heat and simmer until sauce begins to thicken, about 5 minutes. Add salt and pepper to taste. Remove from heat and cover to keep sauce warm.

3. Heat a heavy stovetop grill pan over high heat.

4. Cut each piece of tempeh in half so you have 4 pieces. Brush tempeh generously on both sides with the remaining tablespoon oil and season with salt and pepper.

5. Place tempeh in hot grill pan and cook for 2 minutes on each side, or until heated through. Remove from heat and slice into 1-inch strips.

6. Return sauce to low heat and add tempeh slices until sauce is heated through. Serve immediately.

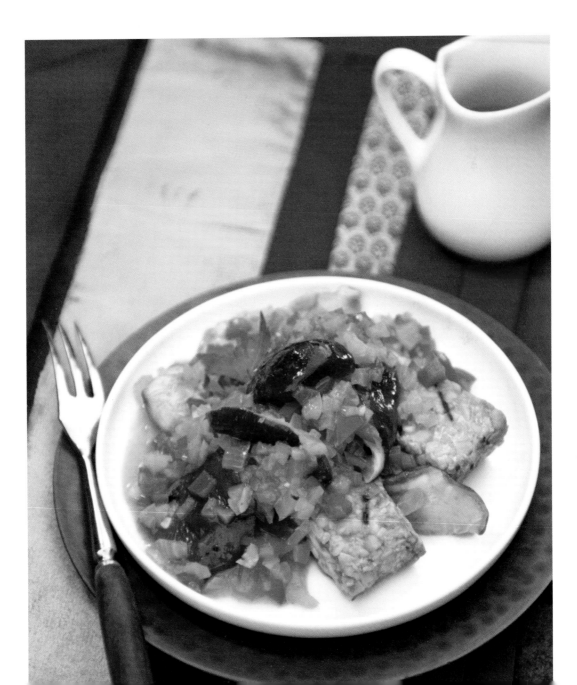

Mariel's Every Season Salad

SERVES 6

Julienne cutters look like vegetable peelers with a deeply serrated edge and are found at cooking supply stores. They make quick work of cutting vegetables!

1 cup peeled and julienned jicama

1 cup peeled and julienned carrots

2 medium tomatoes, cut into wedges

1 cup peeled and julienned roasted red beets

1 cup julienned yellow bell peppers

1 tablespoon fresh lemon juice

3 tablespoons white balsamic vinegar

1 teaspoon sea salt

¼ teaspoon white pepper

5 tablespoons extra light olive oil

1 head limestone or butter lettuce

1. Place jicama, carrots, parsnips, beets, and bell peppers in a bowl and set aside.

2. In another bowl whisk together lemon juice, vinegar, salt, pepper, and olive oil.

3. Drizzle vinaigrette over vegetables. Spoon veggies over lettuce and serve.

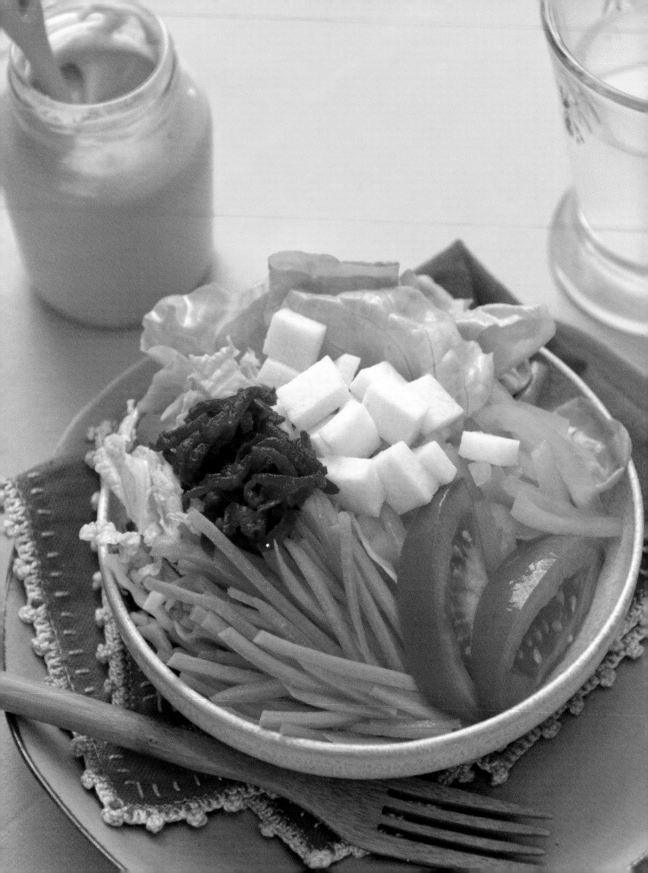

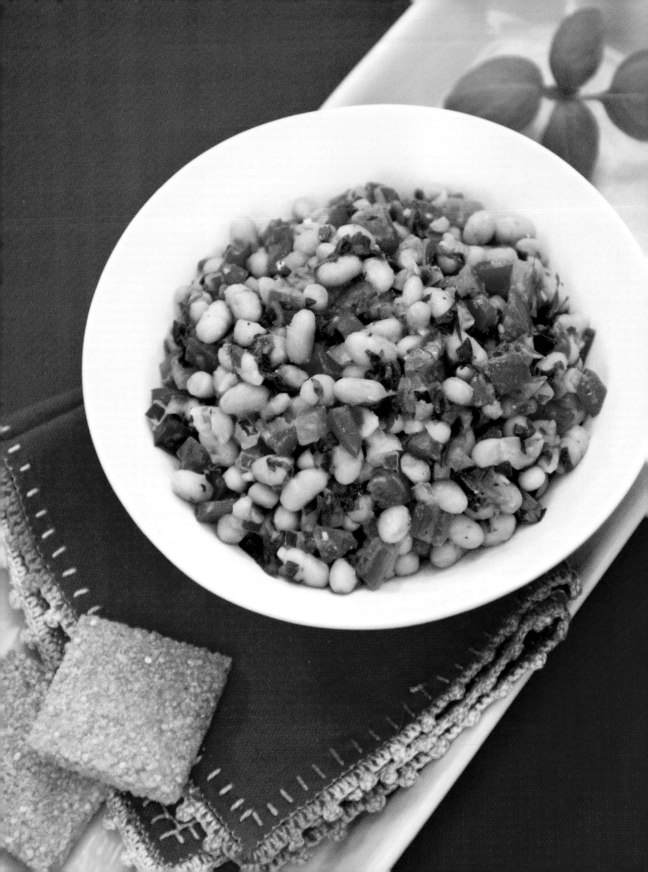

Warm Mediterranean White Bean Salad

SERVES 8

2 (14-ounce) cans white beans, rinsed and drained

2 tablespoons lemon juice

1 tablespoons coconut oil

⅓ cup minced red onion

1 red bell pepper, finely chopped

2 plum tomatoes, finely chopped

1 clove garlic, minced

⅓ cup finely chopped basil leaves

Sea salt

Freshly ground black pepper

1. Place all ingredients in a medium bowl
and toss to combine. Chill until ready to serve.

Replace 1 can of the white beans with black, pinto, or garbanzo beans. Add 2 cups of cooked and crumbled Turkey and Veggie Sausages (pg. 42) to make this a complete meal.

Fiesta Salad

This salad is
wonderful for
lunch or even
brunch.

1 tablespoon coconut or olive oil

1 medium yellow onion, chopped

1 pound organic lean ground turkey

1 teaspoon ancho chile powder

½ teaspoon paprika

¼ teaspoon ground cumin

⅛ teaspoon ground oregano

Salt

Freshly ground black pepper

Pinch of cayenne pepper

1 (15-ounce) can black beans, rinsed and drained

1 large tomato, diced

1 (8-ounce) can organic, low sodium tomato sauce

¼ cup roughly chopped cilantro

1 head romaine lettuce, shredded

1 avocado, peeled, pitted, and diced

4 ounces organic cheddar cheese, shredded (1 cup)

1 (7-ounce) bag baked black bean chips

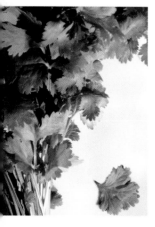

1. Heat oil in a large skillet over medium-high heat. Add onion and
cook, stirring frequently, until soft, about 3 minutes.

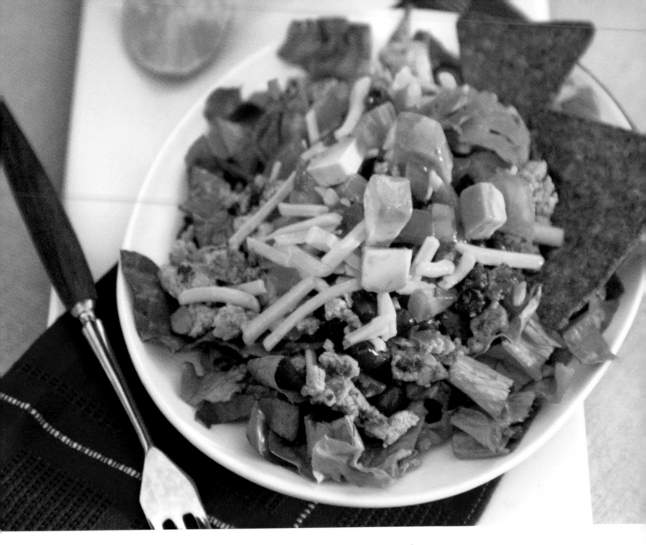

2. Add turkey, ancho chile powder, paprika, cumin, and oregano. Cook, stirring often to break up turkey, until turkey is cooked through, about 5 minutes. Season with salt and pepper to taste.

3. Add black beans, tomato, tomato sauce, and cilantro and cook until heated through.

4. Spoon turkey mixture over romaine lettuce. Garnish with avocado and cheese. Serve with black bean chips.

Fall Vegetable Paella

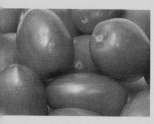

SERVES 6

Garnish with
lemon wedges
if desired. Add
leftover roasted
chicken to
paella for a
nonvegetarian
meal. Substitute
I cup fresh or
frozen (thawed)
organic peas for
edamame, if you
prefer.

1 tablespoon coconut or olive oil

1 small yellow onion, diced

4 cloves garlic, minced

1 medium red bell pepper, diced

6 ounces medium button or
   cremini mushrooms, quartered

2 cups organic vegetable broth

⅛ teaspoon saffron threads

1 teaspoon paprika

½ teaspoon salt

¼ teaspoon cayenne pepper

1 bay leaf

1 ½ cups quick-cooking brown rice

4 fresh plum tomatoes, seeds removed and diced

1 small organic zucchini, cut into ½ inch cubes

6 organic fresh or frozen and thawed
   artichoke hearts, quartered

1 cup organic GMO-free shelled edamame *Regular peas*

1. Add olive oil to a large sauté pan over medium heat. Add onion, garlic, bell pepper, and mushrooms and sauté until onion is soft and mushrooms have given up most of their liquid, stirring often, 5 to 7 minutes. Remove from heat and set aside.

2. In a large saucepan or Dutch oven, bring the broth to a simmer over medium-high heat. Stir in saffron, paprika, salt, cayenne, and bay leaf. Stir in onion mixture, rice, tomatoes, zucchini, and artichoke hearts. Return to a simmer, cover, reduce heat, and cook until rice has absorbed liquid, about 10 minutes.

3. Remove from heat and discard bay leaf. Add edamame and gently fluff with a fork to combine. Cover paella and let sit an additional 5 minutes before serving.

You can also substitute a total of 2 cups of other seasonal vegetables, such as broccoli, cauliflower, carrots, or parsnips in place of artichoke hearts and zucchini.

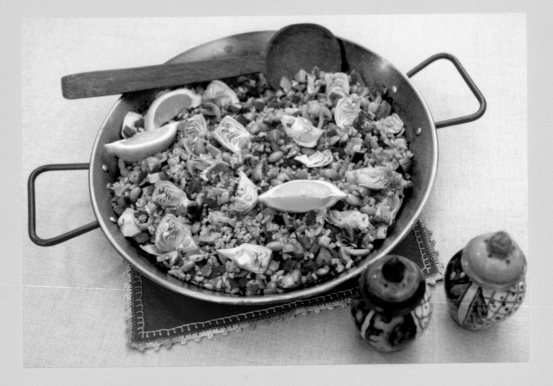

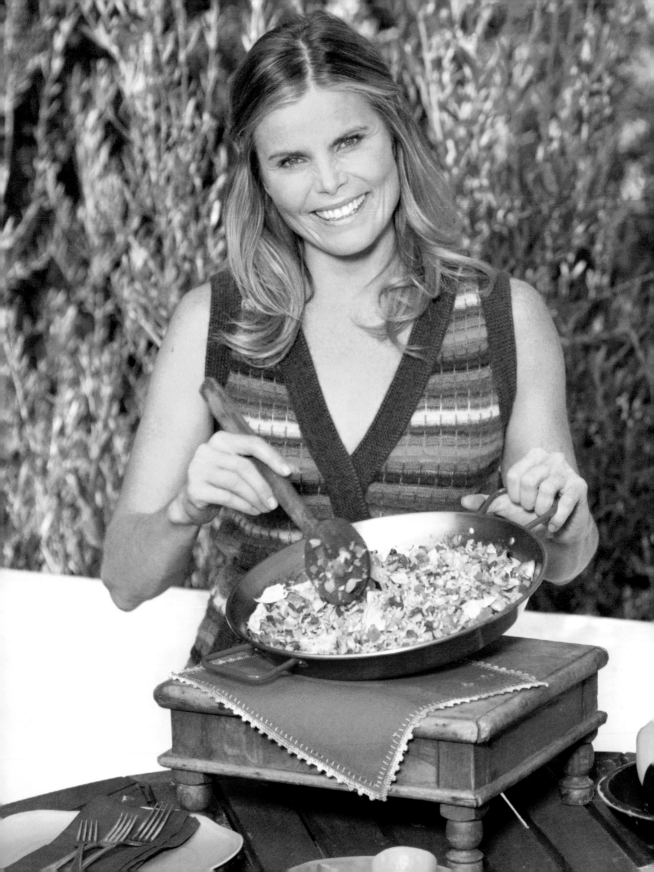

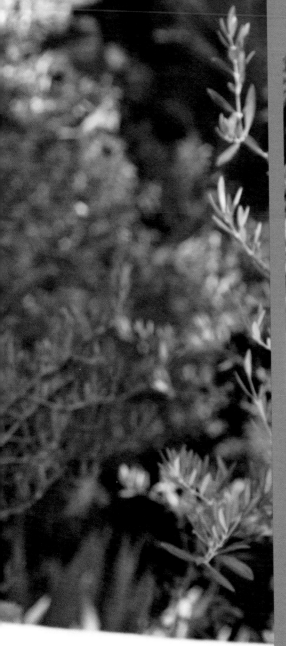

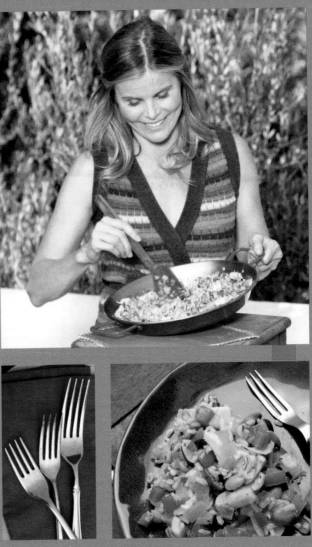

Adapting traditional dishes to make them lighter and healthier is one of my favorite kitchen tricks. Spanish paella is usually loaded with chorizo sausage and seafood; my veggie version is quick, colorful, and practical because it allows for improvisation with whatever produce I have fresh that day.

Buffalo Meatloaf

You can
substitute the
roasted red
pepper and
tomato sauce
with Sugar-Free
Ketchup (pg. 49).

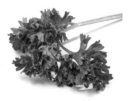

SERVES 6

Coconut or olive oil for greasing loaf pan

1 roasted red bell pepper, diced

½ cup organic low-sodium tomato sauce

2 teaspoons balsamic vinegar

1 teaspoon Xylosweet

1 small onion, diced

2 tablespoons chopped fresh parsley

2 teaspoons chopped fresh thyme

1 ½ pounds ground free-range buffalo meat

2 large eggs, lightly beaten

½ teaspoon sea salt

½ teaspoon freshly ground black pepper

¼ teaspoon dried crushed red pepper

1. Preheat oven to 350°F. Grease a 9-inch or 10-inch loaf pan with a little coconut or olive oil and set aside.

2. Combine half of the red bell pepper, ¼ cup of the tomato sauce, all the vinegar and Xylosweet in the bowl of a mini food processor or blender. Blend until combined but still slightly chunky. Set aside.

3. Combine the remaining half red bell pepper, ¼ cup tomato sauce, all the onion, parsley, thyme, buffalo meat, eggs, salt, pepper, and crushed red pepper in a large mixing bowl and

mix together with clean hands until well combined. Pack into prepared loaf pan and top with tomato sauce mixture.

4. Bake until the internal temperature of the meat reaches 155°F, about 1 hour. Allow loaf to rest at least 15 minutes before slicing.

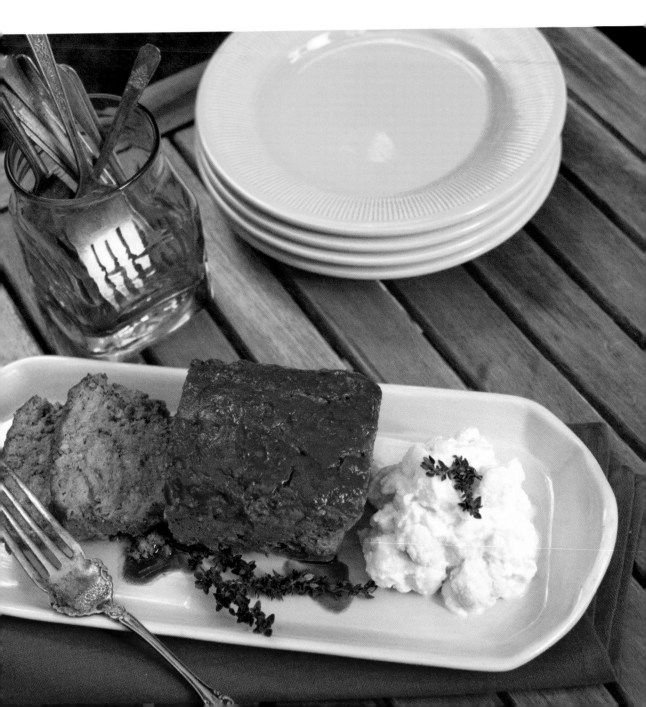

Roasted Chicken with Rosemary and Root Vegetables

SERVES 6-8

There are a number of seasonal root vegetables to choose from. Look for fresh, organic carrots, red and golden beets, celery root, parsnips, fennel bulbs, rutabagas, and turnips in your produce section or farmers' market. Potatoes are also a good addition. Look for fingerling, Yukon gold, small red, or purple potatoes, which are also delicious with this recipe.

¼ cup kosher salt

1 organic free-range roasting chicken, about 6 pounds

3 pounds mixed organic root vegetables, cleaned and peeled

2 large onions peeled, quartered (root end left intact)

1 head garlic, cloves divided, unpeeled

¼ cup olive oil

Sea salt and freshly ground black pepper to taste

⅓ cup chopped fresh rosemary, divided

1 fresh organic lemon, quartered

1. Dissolve ¼ cup kosher salt in 4 cups of cold water in a large stock pot. Rinse chicken inside and out with cold water and add to stock pot. Add enough cold water to completely cover chicken. Cover and let chicken soak in brine for 1 hour. Remove from brine, rinse inside and out and pat dry with paper towels.

2. While chicken is brining, cut root vegetables into 3-inch pieces and place in a large mixing bowl. Add one of the whole quartered onions and all the garlic. Drizzle vegetables with half the olive oil and season with salt, pepper and half of the rosemary. Mix to combine. Set aside.

3. Preheat oven to 375°F.

4. Rub the chicken inside and out with remaining olive oil. Season inside and out with salt, pepper and remaining rosemary. Place lemon and remaining onion inside the cavity. Tuck wings back and under to secure. Tie legs together with butcher twine. Place chicken, breast side down, on roasting rack in a large, heavy roasting pan. Surround chicken with root vegetables and place, uncovered, into oven.

5. Roast for 30 minutes, then turn chicken breast side up. Continue roasting, uncovered, basting with pan juices every half-hour and stirring vegetables occasionally until internal temperature reaches 160°F, or about 2 hours total cooking time, or 20 minutes per pound. (If chicken appears to be browning too quickly, tent with aluminum foil.) Remove from oven and allow meat to rest at least 15 minutes before slicing. Serve with roasted root vegetables on the side.

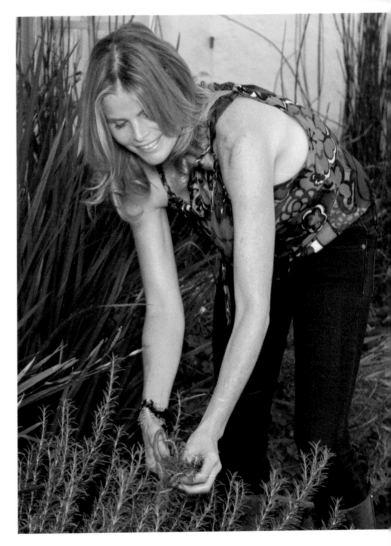

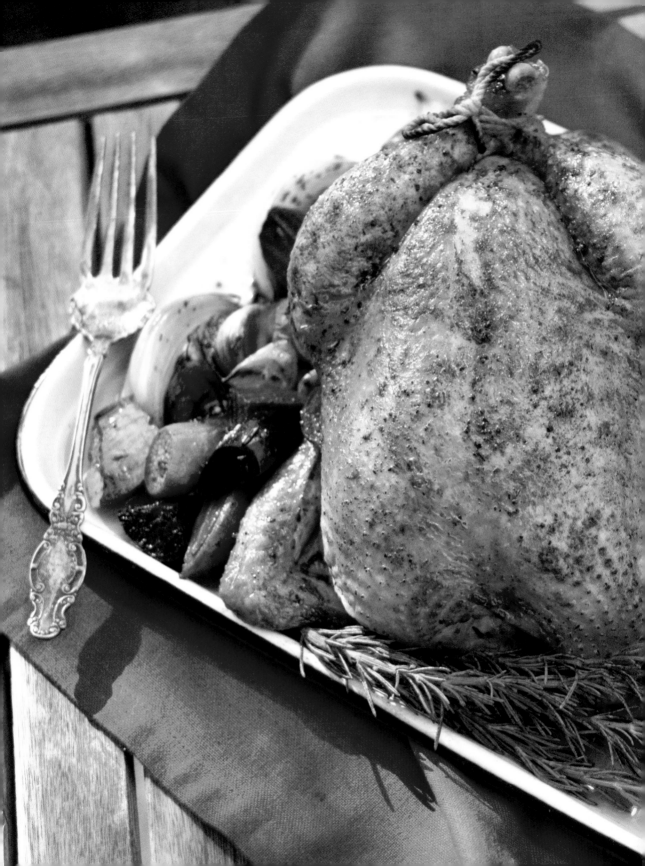

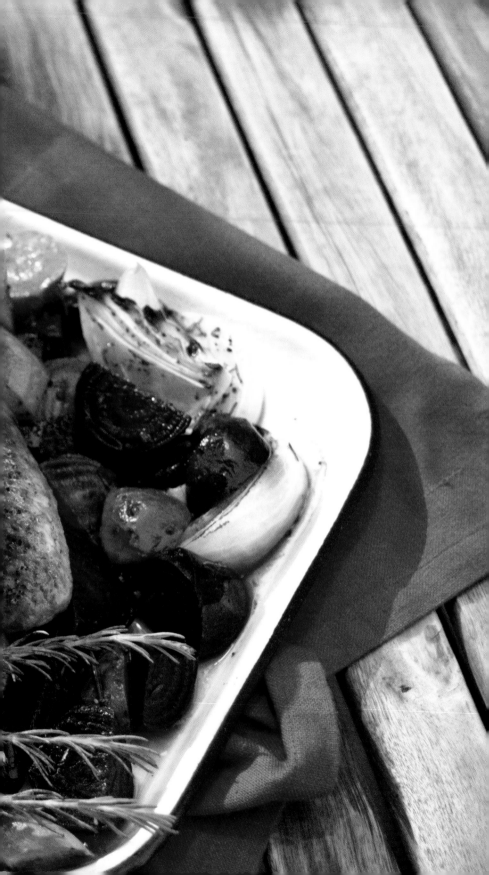

Chocolate Almond Walnut Brownie Cake

A real chocolate lover's cake.

SERVES 8–10

Nonstick cooking spray

8   ounces dark chocolate, chopped

½   cup almond meal

3   tablespoons unsweetened cocoa powder

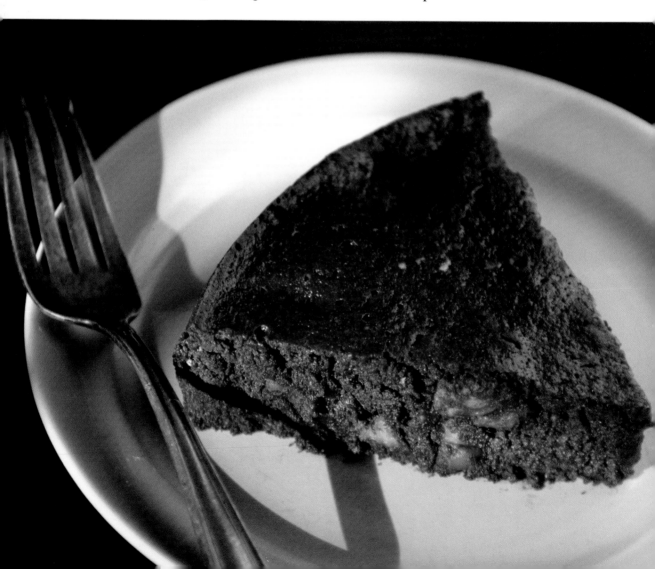

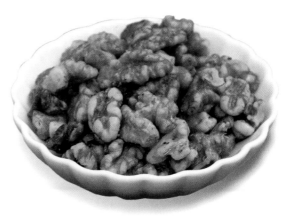

¼	teaspoon baking powder
¼	teaspoon salt
1	cup Xylosweet
5	tablespoons coconut oil
4	large eggs
1 ½	teaspoons vanilla extract
1	cup chopped walnuts

1. Preheat oven to 350°F.

2. Spray an 8-inch springform pan with nonstick cooking spray.

3. Place dark chocolate in a microwave-safe bowl and heat on high at 30 second intervals, stirring between intervals, until chocolate has melted and is smooth. Set aside.

4. In a medium bowl stir together almond meal, cocoa powder, baking powder, and salt.

5. In a separate bowl, using an electric mixer, beat Xylosweet and coconut oil until well combined.

6. Add eggs one at a time to Xylosweet mixture, beating well after each addition. Continue beating until mixture has turned pale and creamy, about 5 minutes.

7. Beat in melted chocolate and vanilla until just blended.

8. Fold in dry ingredients and walnuts.

9. Pour into prepared springform pan and bake until cooked through, about 35 minutes. Let cool before cutting.

Lemon Zest Cheesecake

Serve with fresh
berries for an
amazing dessert.
Cut cheesecake
into small,
bite-size pieces
and freeze for
a creamy sweet
treat anytime.

SERVES 16

Crust:

1 ½ cups Basic Blisscuit dough (pg. 36)

Filling:

Coconut oil for greasing pan

4 (8-ounce) packages goat or sheep's milk cream cheese

1 cup Xylosweet

4 large eggs

1 ½ teaspoons vanilla extract

2 tablespoons lemon zest

1. Preheat oven to 300°F. Rub the bottom and sides of a 9-inch springform pan with coconut oil.

2. Press 1 ¼ cups Basic Blisscuit mix into bottom of prepared pan.

3. Place cream cheese, Xylosweet, eggs, vanilla, and half of the zest in the work bowl of a food processor and process until mixture is smooth. Reserve ¼ cup of the Basic Blisscuit mix for garnishing later.

4. Pour batter into prepared pan and sprinkle with reserved Basic Blisscuit mix. Bake until filling is set in the center, about 1 hour 15 minutes.

5. Allow to cool completely before refrigerating. Let chill for at least 4 hours before serving. Garnish with remaining zest before serving.

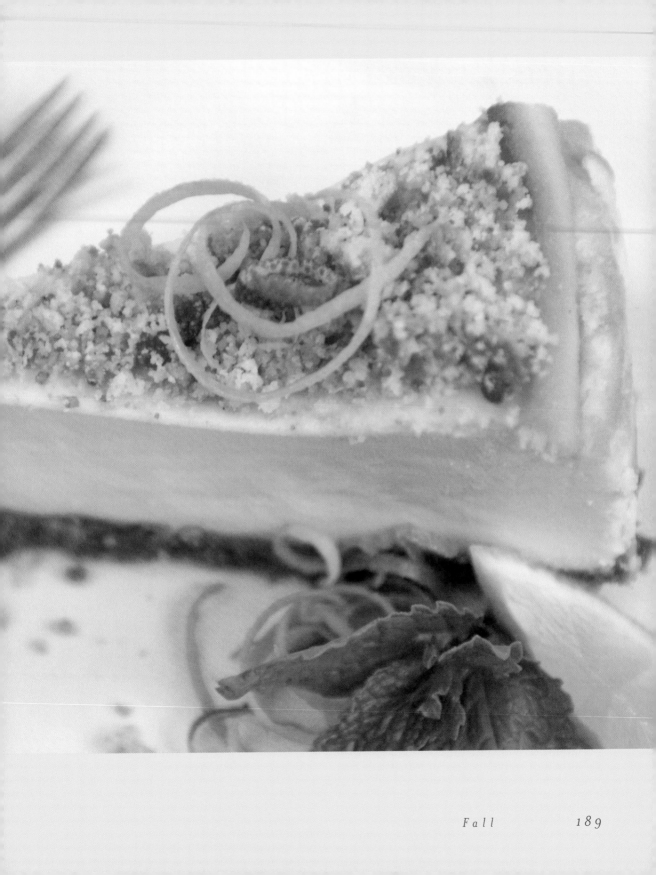

Pumpkin Walnut Balls

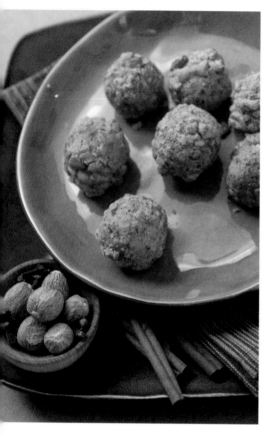

MAKES 2 DOZEN BALLS

2 cups Basic Blisscuit dough (pg. 36)

1 cup organic canned pumpkin

⅓ cup coconut flour

3 ½ tablespoons ground cinnamon

1 cup unsweetened cocoa powder

1 large egg white, lightly beaten

1 cup finely chopped walnuts

1. Preheat oven to 325°F. Cover a baking sheet with parchment paper and set aside.

2. Place Blisscuit dough in a medium bowl and add pumpkin, flour, and cinnamon, stirring to thoroughly combine.

3. Using 1 tablespoon of dough at a time, form dough into balls.

4. Roll each ball in cocoa powder and dust off the excess. Roll each ball in egg whites and then in the walnuts to completely cover.

5. Place each ball on prepared baking sheet, pressing down slightly so they don't roll off, and bake for 20 minutes or until they are cooked all the way through.

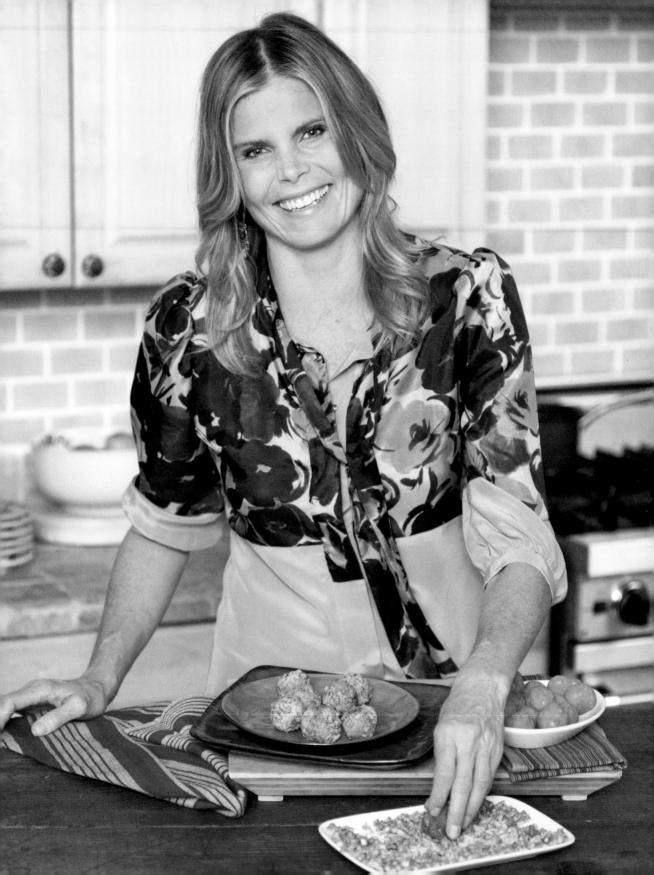

Green Beans Almandine

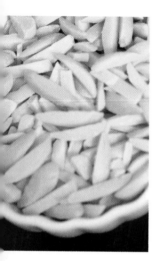

SERVES 4–6

1 pound organic green beans or haricots vert, trimmed

2 tablespoons coconut or almond oil

2 ounces blanched slivered almonds

2 tablespoons chopped flat-leaf parsley

1 teaspoon lemon zest

¼ teaspoon red pepper flakes

Sea salt

Freshly ground black pepper

1. Bring a large pot of salted water to a boil over medium-high heat. Blanch green beans briefly, just until they turn bright green. Drain and run under cold water to stop the cooking. Set aside.

2. Heat oil over medium heat in a large skillet. Add the almonds, parsley, zest, and red pepper flakes. Cook, stirring frequently, until almonds begin to color, 2 to 3 minutes. Add beans to the skillet and cook, stirring often, until cooked through, about 2 minutes. Add salt and pepper to taste. Serve immediately.

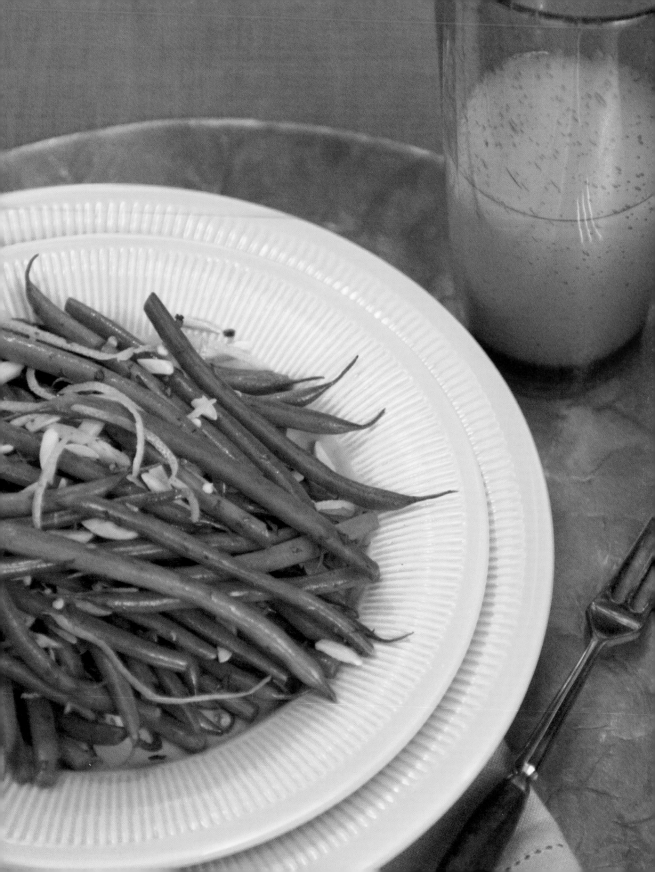

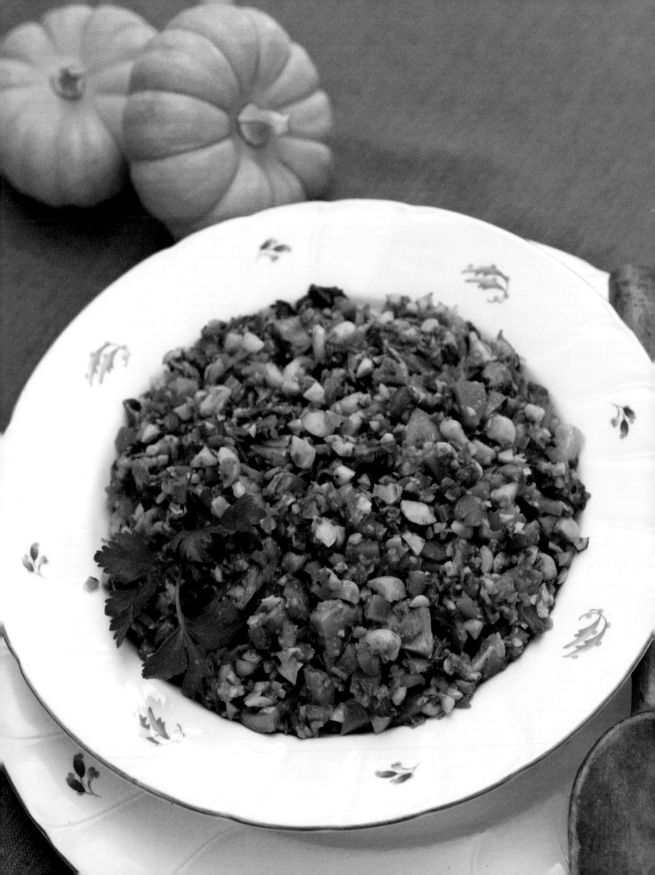

Hazelnut Stuffing with Mushrooms

SERVES 6–8

- 3 tablespoons coconut oil
- 1 small yellow onion, diced
- 2 medium organic carrots, diced
- 2 medium organic celery stalks, diced
- 2 garlic cloves, minced
- 1 ½ pounds medium-size mushrooms, button, cremini, or a mix
- 1 cup hazelnuts, roasted, skins removed, coarsely chopped
- 2 tablespoons chopped fresh sage
- 2 tablespoons chopped fresh parsley
- Sea salt
- Freshly ground black pepper
- 2 large eggs, lightly beaten

add Chestnuts

1. Preheat oven to 350°F. Lightly grease an 8- or 9-inch baking pan with 1 teaspoon of the oil.

2. Heat 1 tablespoon of the oil in a large sauté pan over medium heat. Add onions, carrots, and celery, cooking until onions become soft, about 4 minutes. Add garlic and sauté just until fragrant, about 1 minute. Remove vegetables to a large mixing bowl and set aside.

(continued)

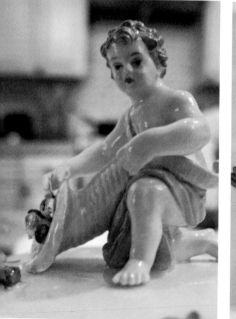

3. Place half of the mushrooms in the bowl of a food processor and coarsely chop. Slice the remaining mushrooms and set aside.

4. Heat 1 tablespoon of the oil in the same sauté pan. Add the coarsely chopped mushrooms and cook until mushrooms have given up most of their liquid, about 5 minutes. Place them in the bowl with the vegetable mixture.

5. Heat the remaining 2 teaspoons oil in the same sauté pan. Add mushroom slices and cook until mushrooms have given up most of their liquid, about 5 minutes. Add to bowl with vegetable mixture.

6. Add hazelnuts, herbs, and beaten eggs to vegetables, stirring to combine. Add salt and pepper to taste. Gently pack mixture into prepared baking pan. Bake until lightly browned, 20 to 25 minutes. Serve warm.

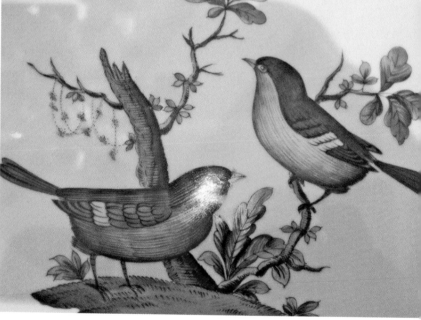

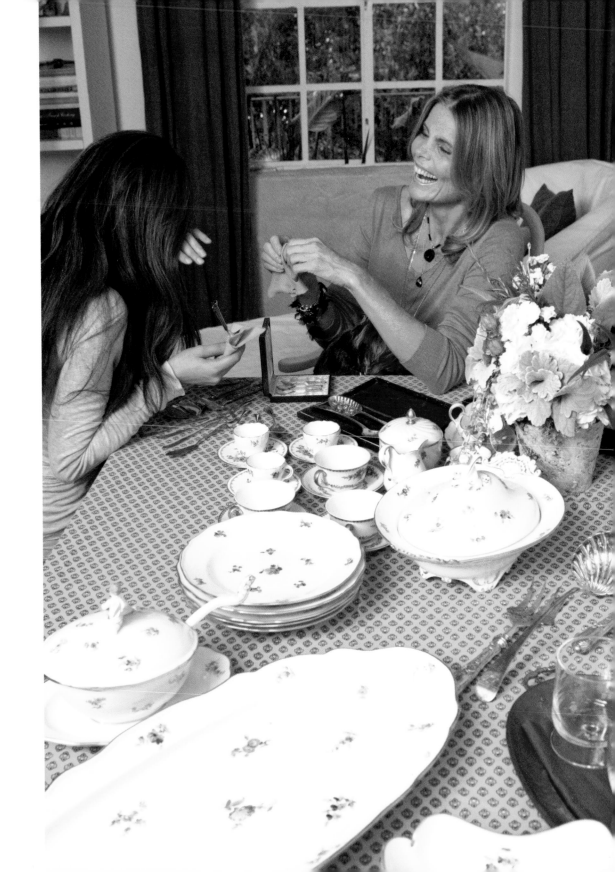

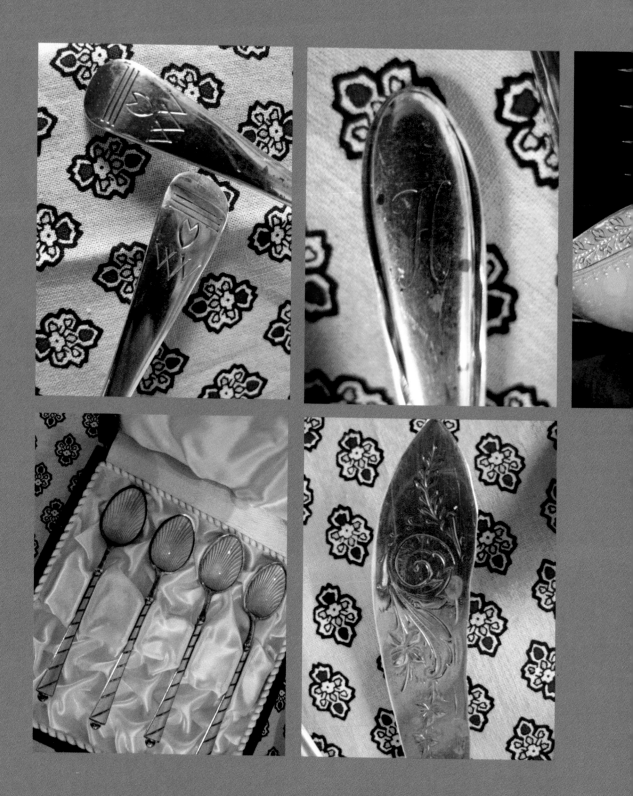

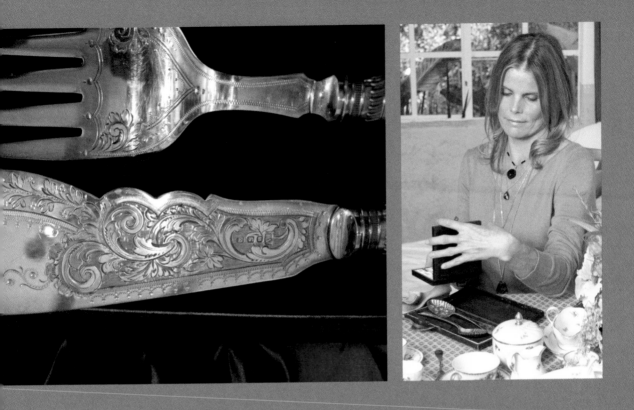

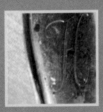

Hemingways always hold a special place for food in our hearts. My grandfather Ernest's silverware is proof of his appreciation for a good meal; my mom's Limoges china tells the story of her own love affair with French cooking. When I use these pieces, or the enameled teaspoons my grandfather collected, it brings a rush of memories to life and connects me to my roots.

Somehow, using the "family china" has come to be seen as old-fashioned or not modern today, but I love to bring it all out as often as possible and not just save it for special occasions. It is fun and joyous to lay a table with these old friends; if you have them, they need to be shared! Collecting vintage pieces of cutlery or chinaware at antique stores or flea markets is a great way to make your own eclectic and personal set—they don't have to be precious, they should just appeal to your senses and individual style. It's something that adds volumes to the rituals of eating together and serving food to those you love.

Shopping

In a perfect world my food would come from an organic garden, a family of chickens, and pastures of happy animals outside my door, because food raised or grown outside of intensive agriculture has more nutrients, fewer chemicals, and is kinder all round. Until that materializes, I try to make the best shopping choices I can. Here is what I look for day to day.

Vegetables

Farmers' market shopping is a preference, as most products are organic *and* local, or at least pesticide-free, meaning the produce has not been sprayed,

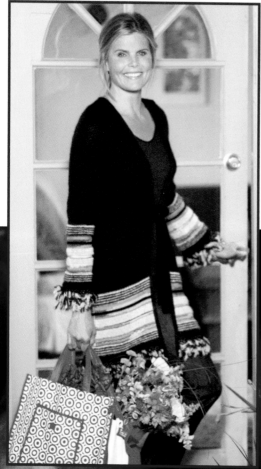

but hasn't yet achieved its organic certification. However, relying on a once-weekly market is not always possible or practical. When shopping at the grocery store, I see if any produce is labeled "locally grown" because it will have been picked riper, which means it will have greater nutritional value and taste. If it's not organic, I soak it for twenty minutes in a sink of cold water with one tablespoon of bleach, then soak it for twenty minutes in a sink of fresh water. This significantly helps reduce pesticides and pathogenic bacteria. I always buy organic green leafy vegetables and berries; these suck up pesticides more than dense or thick-skinned produce.

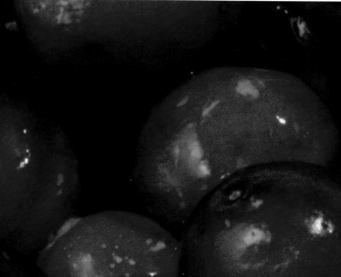

Eggs

The labeling on eggs is confusing and for good reason: most egg production, even if cage free and organic, involves intensive farming methods. At the supermarket, those eggs are still the better bet. (Free range doesn't actually guarantee the hens had better treatment.) Finding pasture-raised eggs on sale at a farm stand or small health-food store is an extra treat. The chickens were allowed to roam free, eat grass and insects, and their eggs have much higher vitamin D and A and omega-3 levels, with lower cholesterol. Sometimes I can find a Certified Humane label on supermarket eggs; this validates they came from higher-grade sources.

Chicken

Organic, free-range chicken is inevitably more expensive than the standard supermarket fare we all grew up with. It's worth it. Eating protein that is free of hormones, antibiotics, and pesticide residues is one of the smartest things we can do. When possible I buy pasture-raised chicken from a local farm and am astonished by the flavor and texture. I eat chicken in moderation.

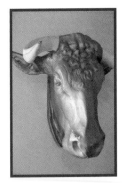

Meat

Less quantity, more quality: I always purchase organic and grass-fed red meat. It is much healthier, with lower fat and higher essential nutrients. I'd rather make a stew with inexpensive, grass-fed chuck than eat a conventional, corn-fed tenderloin. I enjoy buying meat from small family farms that ship frozen meat to the door. The animals are raised responsibly and ethically under top quality control with no antibiotics or hormones. This is not as expensive as it may seem, if you use meat sparingly and deliberately. The benefits to body and planet are huge.

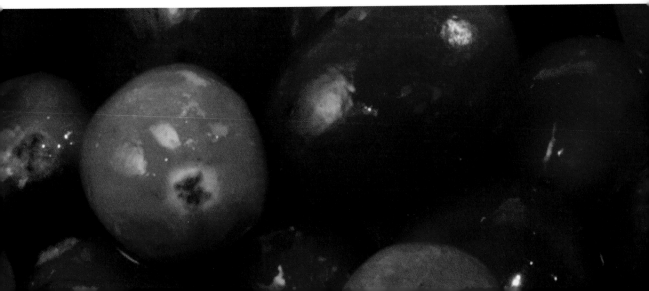

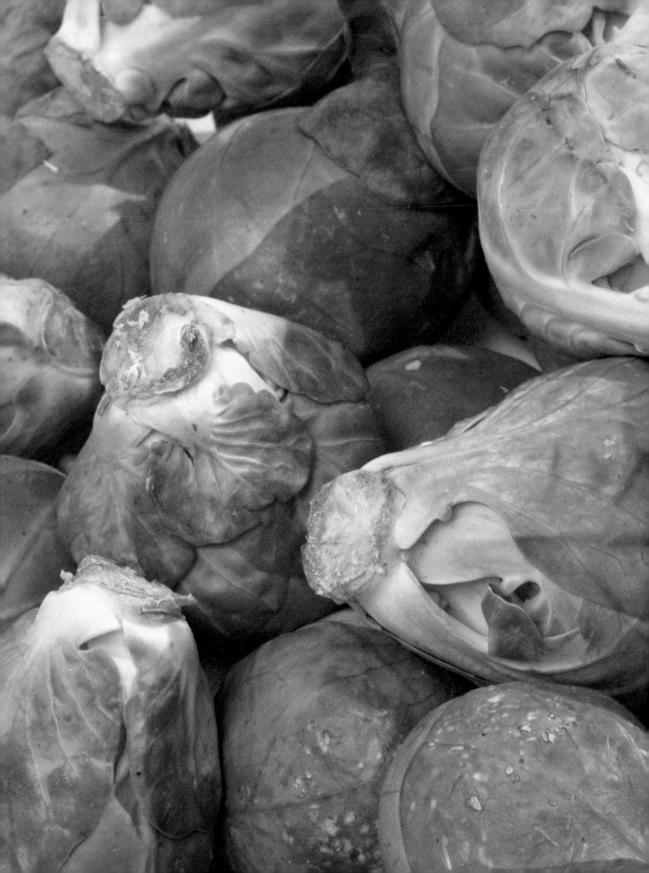

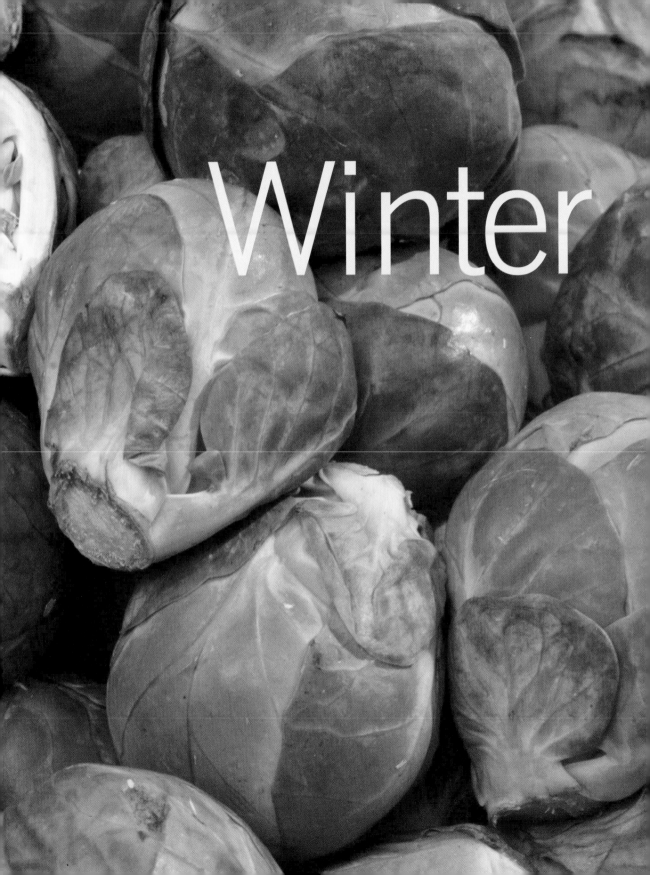

Winter

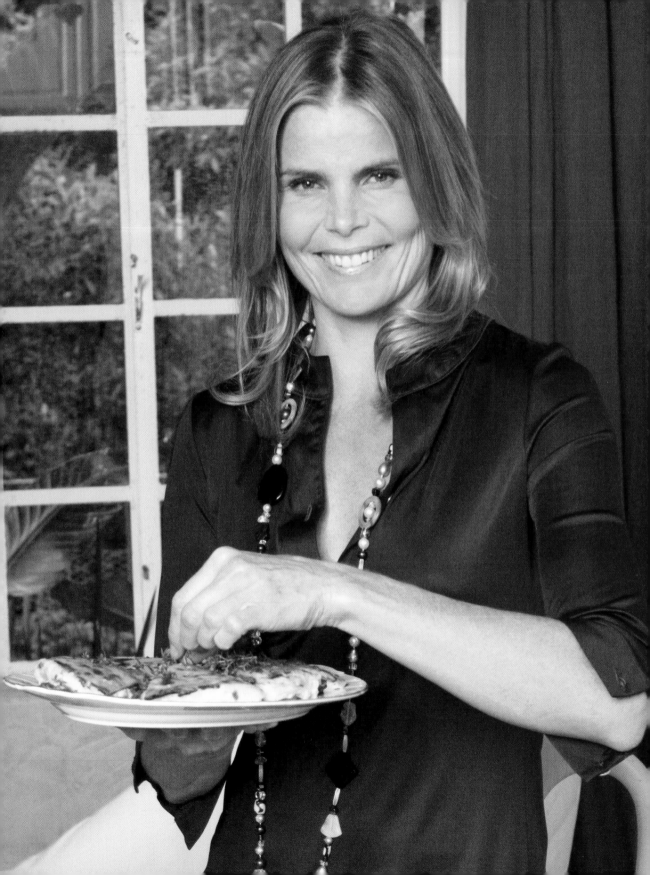

Cozy, Healthy, Comfort Foods

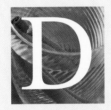**D**eep reds, rich browns, and my favorite food color, purple, find their way into my saucepans and serving bowls as the winter rolls on. Those are the shades of my cold-weather comfort meals and they reflect the changing scenery outside my canyon home. The giant trees have turned from green to gold, and as I drive home over the twisty, mountain road, the sky turns indigo-gray. Returning from city duties to enjoy Roasted Tomato Soup, or better still the Grass-Fed Pot Roast with Wild Mushrooms and Cipollini Onions, cooked for hours with one of my daughters doing the braising, feels just about right. In winter, we instinctively seek out foods that warm and nurture.

For some people the idea of soupy, stew-like foods is all too boring. Maybe they were fed too much bland chicken-noodle from a can in their youth. They're going to miss out on the joyous secret to anything pureed, mashed, or cooked in one pot: it makes meals so easy. Plus, when you're committed to cooking fresh, and you play with herbs and spices, steaming bowls explode with flavor. *Fresh* may seem a counterintuitive instruction, given the closed-up state of nature. But look closely around—nature's still alive; it's just less splashy. The stuff on sale similarly may seem a little ordinary, but it's hardy and full of potential. Instead of relying exclusively on shipped-in and frozen produce during the winter, recognize the season as a great time to keep cooking with local, seasonal ingredients.

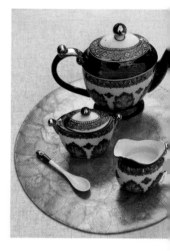

This season's beauty is more subtle.

Onions, rarely celebrated, are grown almost everywhere year-round. They are the center point of a whole family of vegetables that includes garlic, leeks, and chives. These pungent plants come alive with delectable flavor when cooked! (Just ask the French about their famous onion soup.) Leeks, the most subtle, are delicious when sautéed as a side—try adding some pancetta and chickpeas for a tasty side dish. Here I use them for a creamy, low-fat soup that takes no time to prepare. (Make soups in big batches and then freeze in small containers to provide for several meals. It may not be as fresh as same-day cooking, but as a replacement for packaged, preserved products, it's still great for you, for your wallet, and for the environment.) Small cipollini onions cook to soft perfection alongside the pot roast; three hours later they melt in

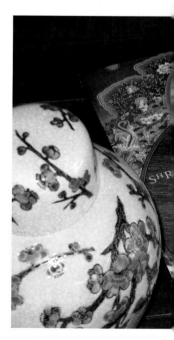

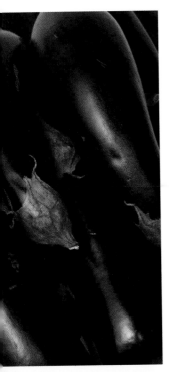

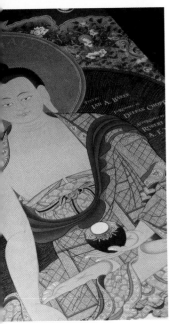

your mouth. And garlic and chives are what make my cauliflower mash one of those things I want to eat every day.

Cauliflower deserves a whole paragraph of its own since I use it so much. It's a substantial, chunky vegetable that provides oomph, is loaded with anti-cancer agents, and can replace starchy potato in many a dish. Eaten raw or steamed without oil, its appeal can be elusive. But turned into a soup or a mash, with the right flavoring, it's a true heart-warmer: thick, soft, and comforting, like sophisticated baby food. When I can find them, I buy purple cauliflowers, because spooning up a bowl of lavender-colored puree that's good for you is surely one of the great joys of dinner. The added bonus is that kids go crazy for it.

This segment is not all about virtuous, savory foods. It's great to have something sweet on chilly mornings and you don't need sugars and syrups, or packaged breakfast products to do it. If a long hike with the dogs is planned, I make my version of oatmeal, Hot Cinnamon Quinoa Mush. This grain gets my vote for its health benefits, but really, I love it for the texture and the flavor when mixed with warm almond milk. Pancakes and waffles can also be wheat and sugar free. The buckwheat in the waffles is not a grain but a fruit seed, and it gives them some heft. Then choose how to top them. Raw butter tastes sensational and is nutrition-ally powerful, if you can find it. Small amounts of raw honey are prized in many health traditions as almost a tonic. I prefer that to agave, the newly popular sweetener made from cacti that is low on the glycemic index but still high in fructose.

Purple shows up again in winter desserts. Pear Sorbet with Balsamic Port Syrup has a jewel-colored, port-wine reduction—the alcohol is burned off and the final syrup is divine. Indigo is also the color of bubbling-hot berries under a crisp top, a cozy supper must-have that takes minimal effort to prepare. (Try a variation with three kinds of apple, topped with a splash of organic heavy cream.) I've baked with many sugar substitutes, and Xylosweet (see Pantry Essentials) works best because it liquefies like sugar on heating.

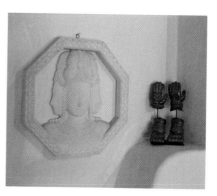

With winter come holiday parties to host and to attend. Serving creative alternatives to boozy drinks and high-fat snacks, or taking some as a gift when I go, makes me happier and lighter, in body *and* spirit. At my house, the Goat-Cheese Tartlets and Baked Sweet Potato Sticks are gone within minutes, so now I quadruple the recipes. It's exactly what you want to see as the dark night draws in around you: people talking and laughing with your simple treats in hand.

Winter's early nightfall can make cooking for the week ahead a nurturing act, not just a necessary job.

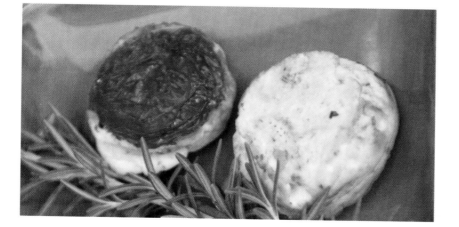

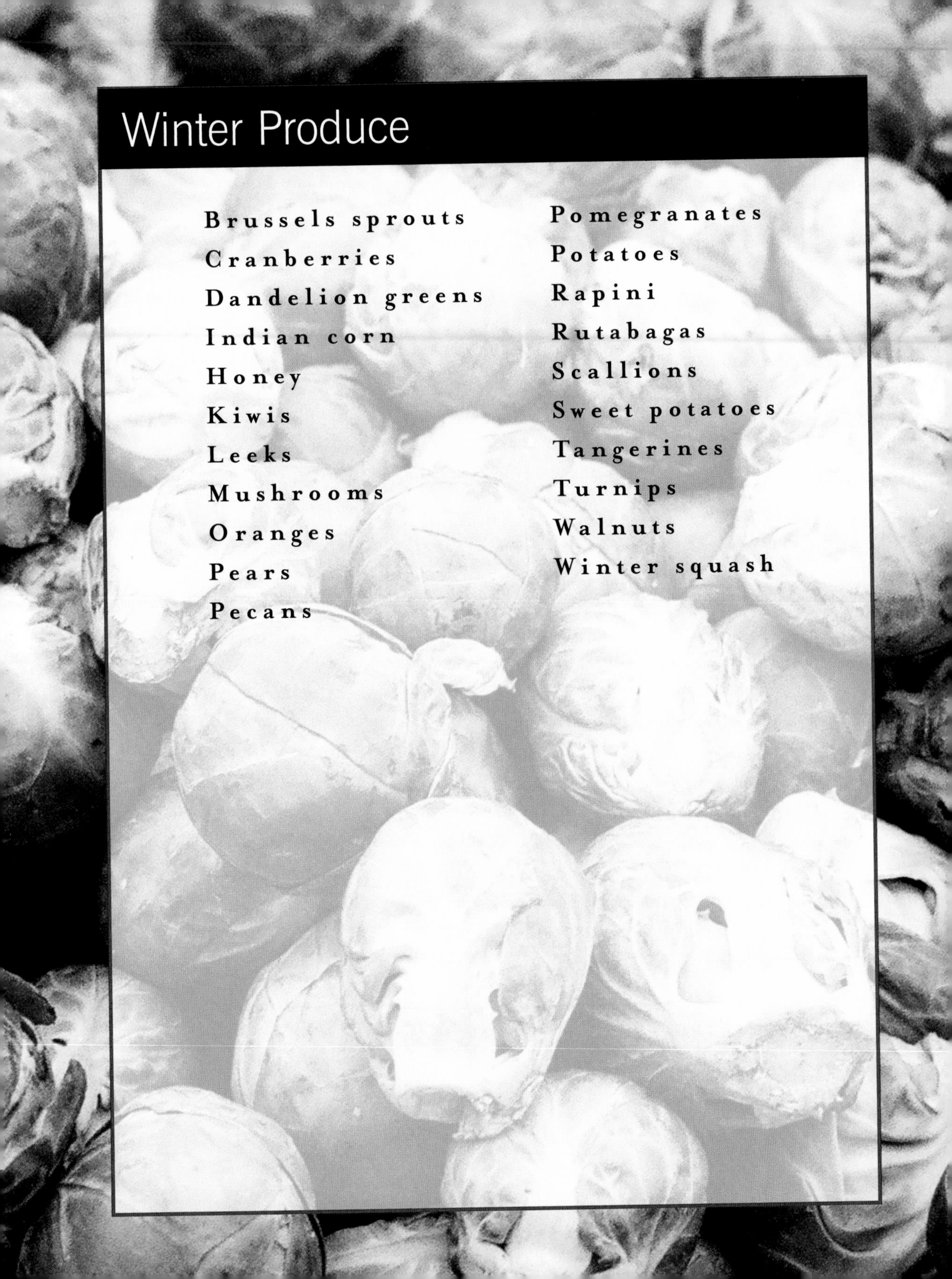

Winter Produce

Brussels sprouts
Cranberries
Dandelion greens
Indian corn
Honey
Kiwis
Leeks
Mushrooms
Oranges
Pears
Pecans

Pomegranates
Potatoes
Rapini
Rutabagas
Scallions
Sweet potatoes
Tangerines
Turnips
Walnuts
Winter squash

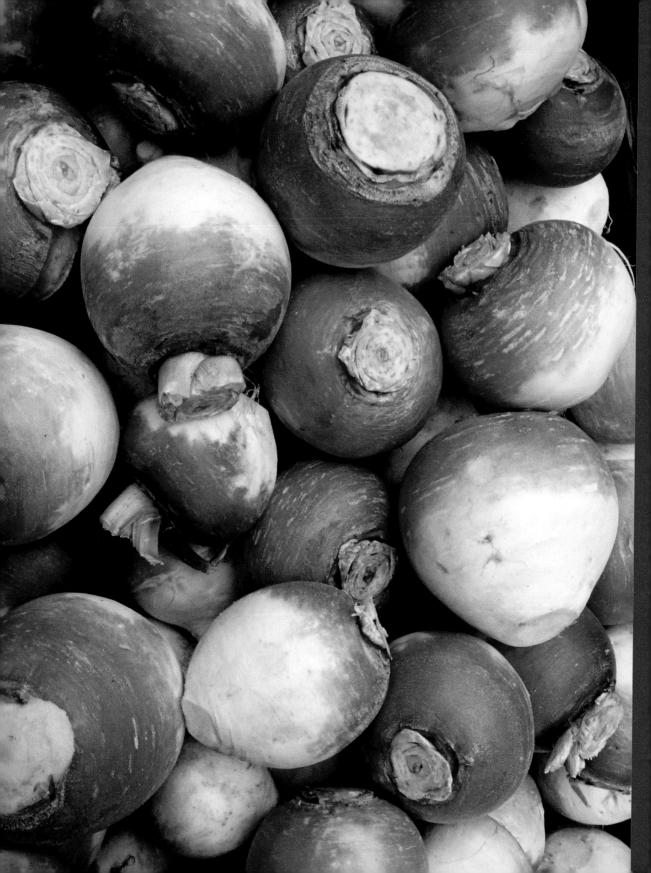

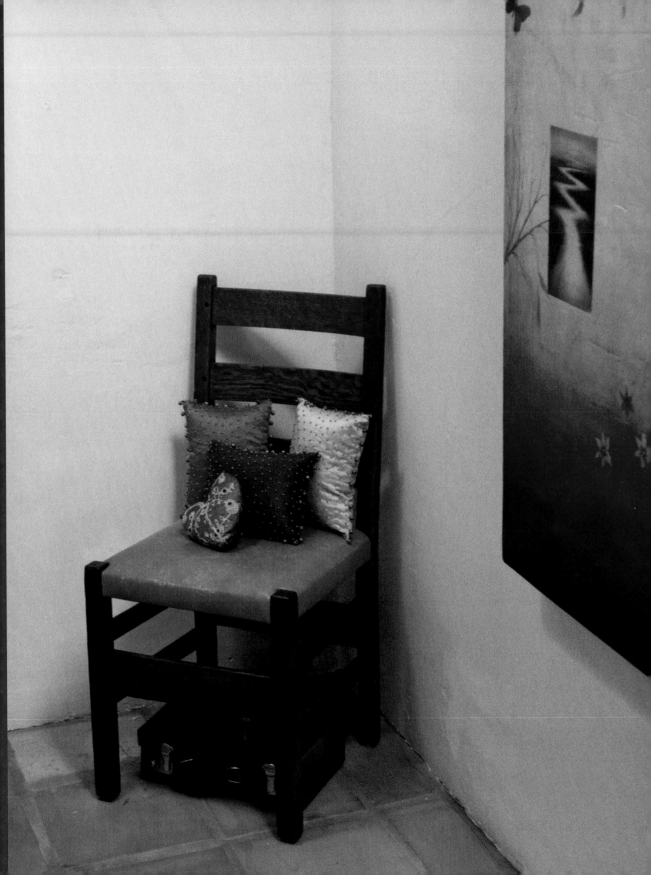

Hot Cinnamon Quinoa Mush

SERVES 6

2 cups rolled oats

I cup coarse ground quinoa

3 tablespoons Xylosweet *Brown sugar or Maple syrup*

3 ½ cups fat-free milk or almond milk

2 teaspoons ground cinnamon, plus more for garnish

1. Place oats, quinoa, Xylosweet, milk, and cinnamon in a medium saucepan.

2. Bring to a gentle simmer and cook, stirring very frequently, until thick and creamy, about 8 minutes.

3. Remove from heat, separate into individual bowls, and garnish with cinnamon.

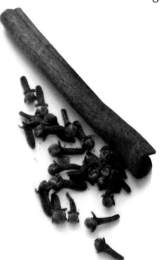

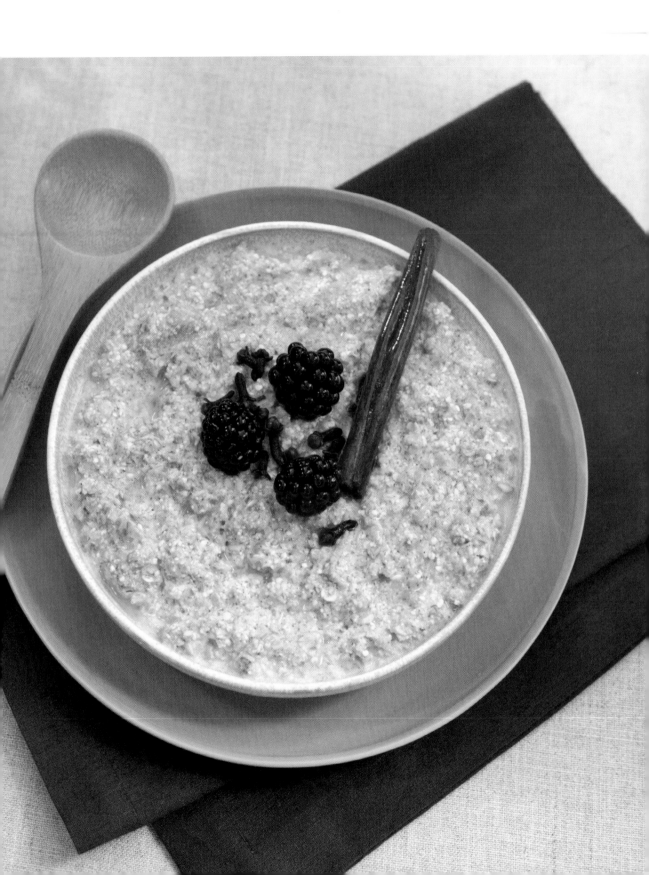

Blueberry Pancakes

SERVES 4

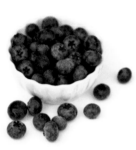

1 tablespoon mascarpone cheese or chèvre cheese

1 teaspoon vanilla extract

½ teaspoon ground cinnamon

¾ cup egg whites

1 tablespoon coconut oil

¾ cup blueberries

1. In a small bowl, using an electric mixer, beat cheese with vanilla and cinnamon until light and fluffy, about 3 minutes. Set aside.

2. In a medium bowl, beat egg whites until stiff peaks begin to form, about 4 minutes.

3. Gently fold cheese mixture into egg whites until just combined.

4. Heat a nonstick skillet on medium-high heat, brushing the pan with oil.

5. Pour about ⅓ cup of batter at a time into pan and cook until edges begin to brown slightly and bubbles begin to appear near the center. Sprinkle with 2 tablespoons of blueberries and fold in half. Cover, lower heat, and let cook for another minute to cook through.

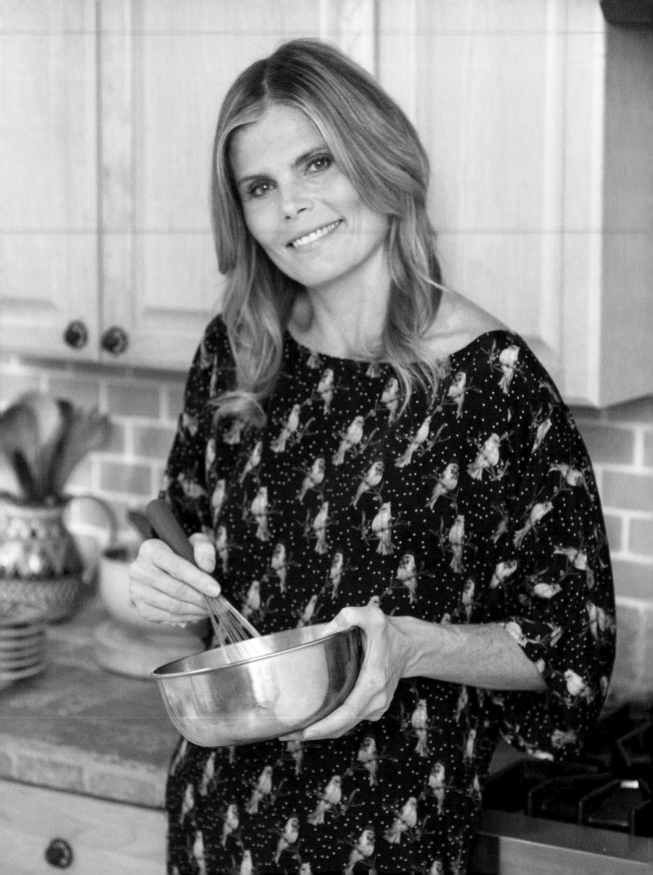

Buckwheat and Coconut Flour Waffles

MAKES ABOUT 8 WAFFLES

½ cup buckwheat flour

½ cup coconut flour

¼ teaspoon sea salt

1 ½ teaspoons baking powder

2 tablespoons Xylosweet

3 large eggs, beaten

1 tablespoon coconut oil, melted

2 cups buttermilk

1. Preheat waffle iron.

2. Mix all ingredients in a medium bowl to combine. Ladle onto hot waffle iron. Cook until golden brown. Serve warm with fresh fruit.

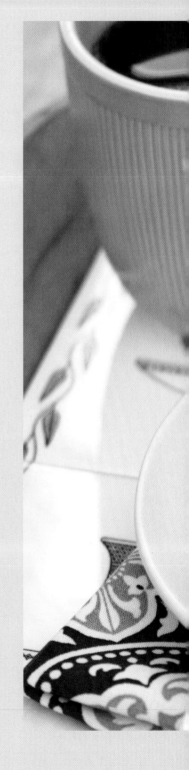

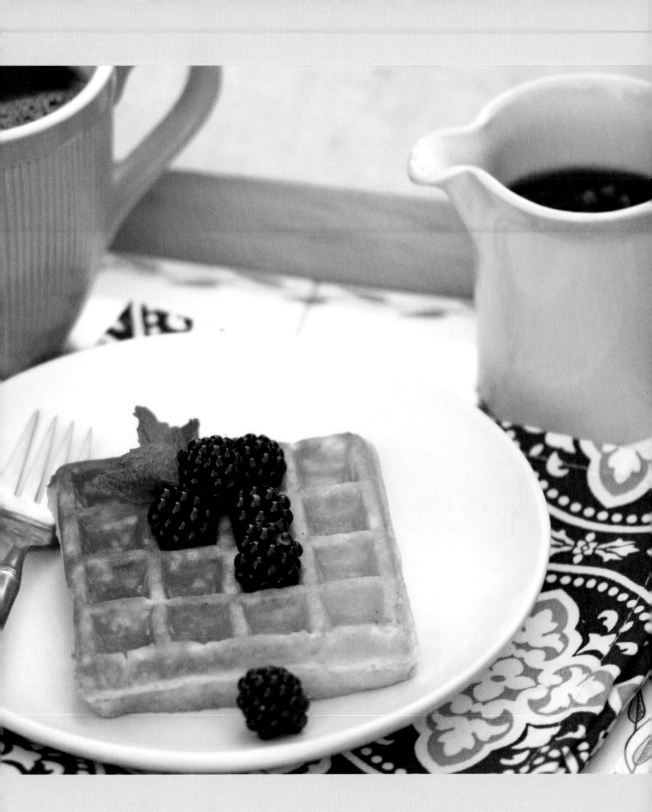

Roasted Tomato Soup

Serve with a
Savory Cheese
Blisscuit
(pg. 38).

SERVES 6

1 pound tomatoes, cut in half

2 garlic cloves, smashed

1 tablespoon coconut oil

   Salt

   Pepper

2 cups organic vegetable stock

¼ cup flat-leaf parsley

2 tablespoons basil

1. Preheat oven to 450°F.

2. Place tomatoes, garlic, and oil in a shallow baking dish
   and toss to coat. Sprinkle with salt and pepper and roast
   for 10 minutes.

3. Place tomatoes, stock, and herbs in the work bowl of a food
   processor and process until smooth.

4. Pour mixture into a medium saucepan
   and bring to a simmer
   to heat through
   before serving.

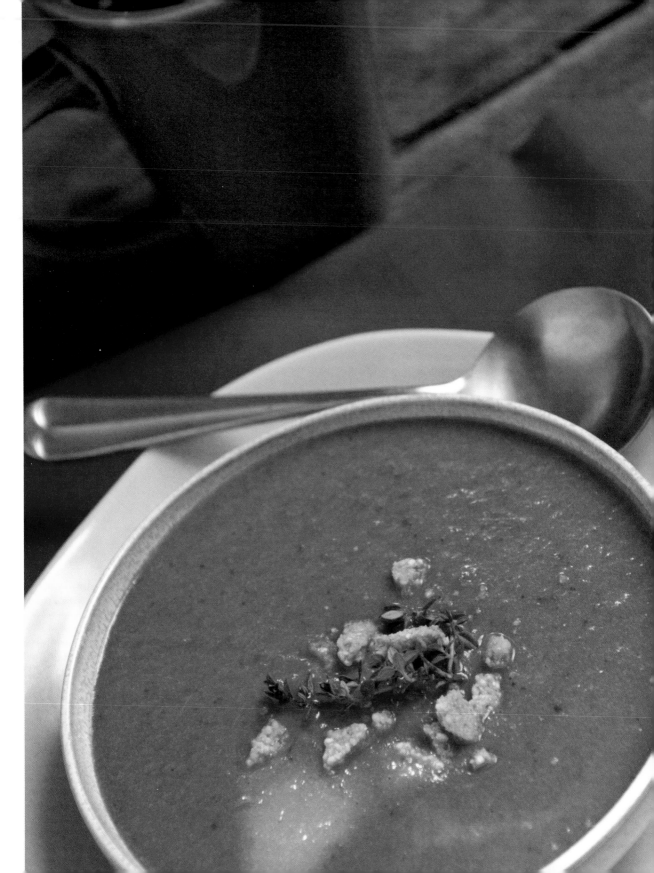

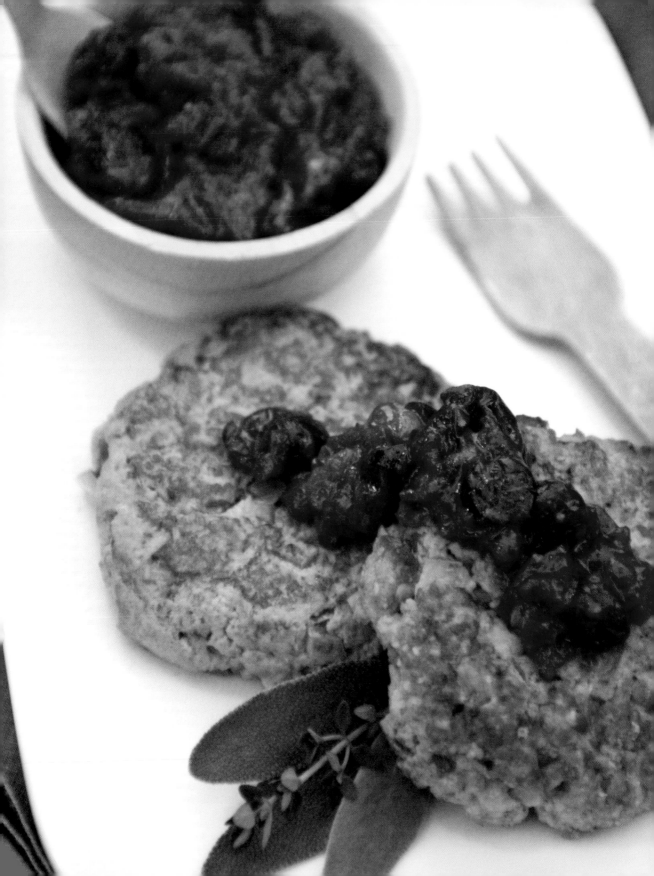

Turkey Burger with Cranberry Sauce

SERVES 4

If fresh cranberries are not available, substitute organic frozen cranberries, thawed. These burgers are great served on top of salad greens.

Cranberry Sauce:

- 1 tablespoon coconut oil
- ½ red onion, diced
- 1 tablespoon minced ginger
- 3 tablespoons orange zest
- 10 ounces fresh cranberries
- 1 cup orange juice
- 2 tablespoons Xylosweet

  Sea salt

  Freshly ground black pepper

Turkey Burgers:

- 1 pound organic free-range ground turkey breast
- ½ small red onion, minced
- 1 clove garlic, minced
- ½ teaspoon organic orange zest
- 1 tablespoon minced sage
- 1 teaspoon minced thyme
- ¼ teaspoon dried red pepper flakes
- 1 large egg, beaten
- 1 tablespoon oil

(continued)

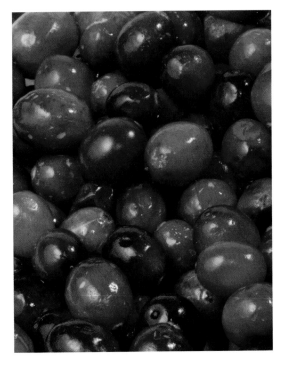

1. To prepare the sauce, heat oil in a medium saucepan over medium heat. Sauté onions, ginger, and zest until onions are soft, 3 to 4 minutes. Add cranberries, orange juice, and Xylosweet. Season to taste with salt and pepper. Bring mixture to a boil, and then reduce heat and simmer until cranberries are very soft and sauce has thickened, about 40 minutes. Can be served warm or cold. Can be stored, covered and refrigerated, for up to a week.

2. To prepare turkey burgers, combine all burger ingredients, except the oil, in a large mixing bowl. Form mixture into 4 patties. Heat oil in a nonstick skillet over medium heat. Cook patties, turning once, until golden brown on both sides and cooked through, about 5 minutes per side.

3. Serve burgers topped with cranberry sauce.

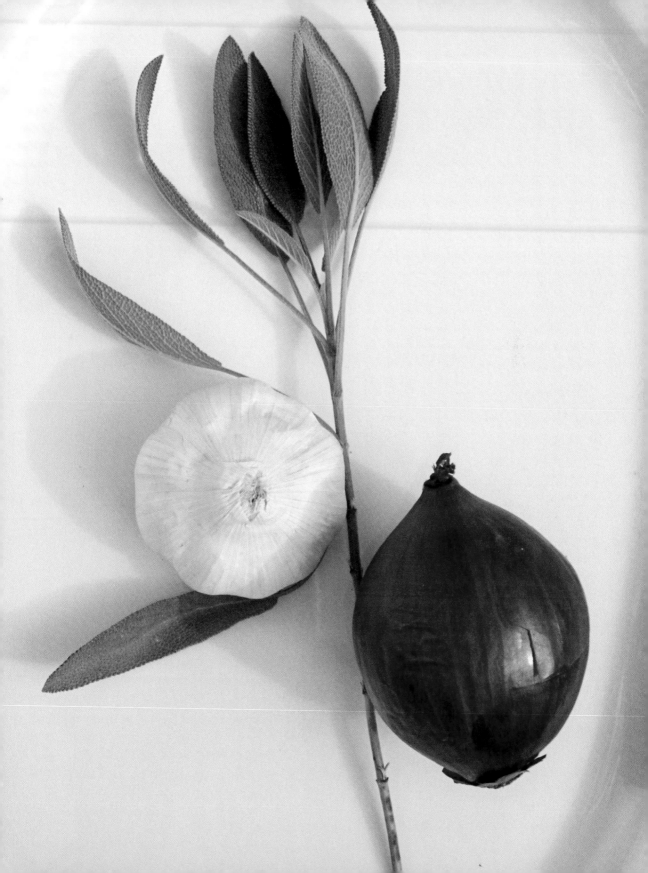

Cauliflower, Leek, and Chèvre Jack Cheese Soup

SERVES 4

If you are
unable to find
a chèvre jack-
style cheese, you
can substitute
a chèvre white
cheddar-style
cheese, or a cow's
milk jack or
white cheddar.

- 1 tablespoon olive oil
- 1 large leek, white and light green part only, thinly sliced
- 2 medium organic carrots, chopped
- 2 medium organic celery stalks, chopped
- 2 garlic cloves, minced
- 1 teaspoon finely chopped thyme
- 1 pound cauliflower florets, chopped
- 4 cups quality organic vegetable or chicken broth
- 4 ounces chèvre jack-style cheese, shredded

  Sea salt

  Freshly ground black pepper

1. Heat oil in a large, heavy pot over medium heat. Add leeks, carrots, and celery and sauté until soft, about 4 minutes. Add garlic and thyme and cook for 2 minutes. Add cauliflower and broth, bring to a boil, and then reduce heat and simmer until cauliflower is very tender, about 15 minutes.

2. Puree mixture in the work bowl of a food processor or blender. Return to pot over very low heat. Add cheese and continue cooking just until cheese melts. Season with salt and pepper. Serve immediately.

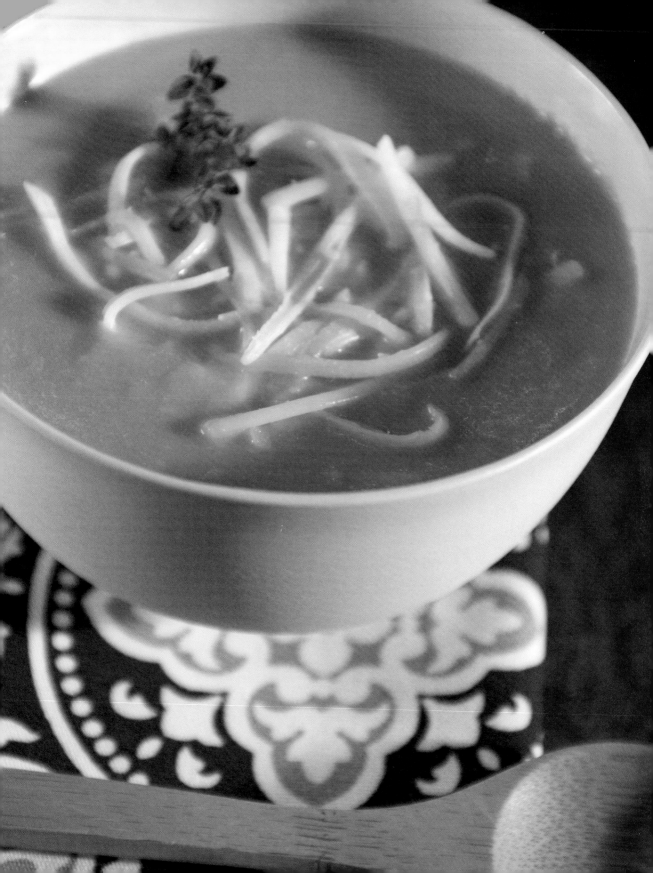

Grass-Fed Beef Pot Roast with Wild Mushrooms and Cipollini Onions

SERVES 6

- 2 tablespoons coconut oil
- 1 boneless grass-fed beef chuck roast, tied (about 3 pounds)
  Sea salt
  Freshly ground black pepper
- 8 ounces small whole cipollini onions, peeled
- ¼ cup balsamic vinegar
- 2 cups low-sodium tomato juice
- 2 cups organic low-sodium beef broth
- 2 bay leaves
- 10 ounces fresh wild mushrooms

1. Preheat oven to 300°F.

2. Heat oil in a large Dutch oven over medium-high heat. Season meat on all sides with salt and pepper and sear until evenly browned on all sides. Remove meat from pan. Add onions and sauté until golden brown. Remove from pan.

3. Add balsamic vinegar to pan, stirring to scrape up any browned bits on the bottom of the pan. Add tomato juice, broth, and

bay leaves and bring to a boil. Then reduce heat and simmer. Add meat, onions, and mushrooms to sauce. Remove from heat, cover, and place in oven. Cook, basting every 30 minutes with the pan juices, until the beef falls apart easily, 2 ½ to 3 hours. Before serving, remove and discard bay leaves.

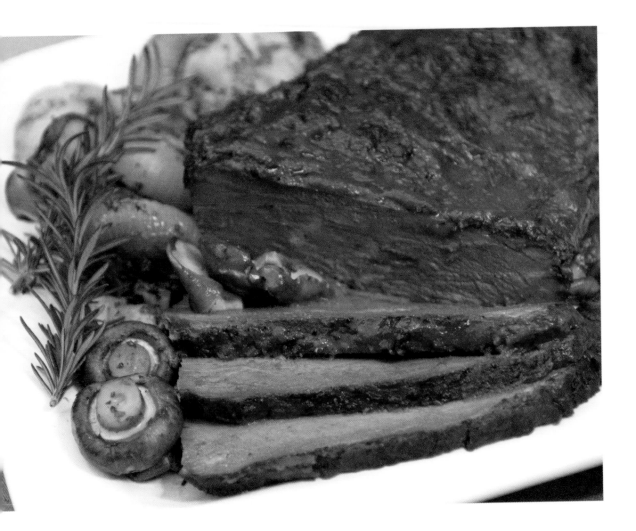

Garlic and Chive
Mashed Cauliflower

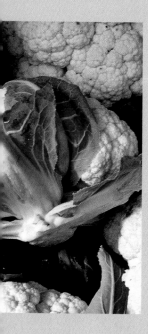

SERVES 4

1   head garlic

     Olive oil for drizzling

1   pound organic cauliflower florets

1   tablespoon unsalted butter

2   tablespoons chopped fresh chives

1. Preheat oven to 400°F.

2. Cut off top of garlic head to expose cloves. Place on a piece
   of foil big enough to form an envelope around the garlic.
   Drizzle with olive oil and enclose in foil. Roast until very
   tender and lightly browned, about 30 minutes. Cool slightly
   before squeezing out cloves and smashing them.

3. Bring a large pot of water with a steamer basket to boil over
   medium-high heat. Steam cauliflower until it is very tender,
   about 5 to 7 minutes. Remove cauliflower to a large mixing
   bowl and mash with a fork to reach desired consistency.
   (For a smoother consistency, add half or all of the cauliflower
   to the bowl of a food processor and process until smooth.
   Return to mixing bowl before continuing.)

4. Add peeled and smashed roasted garlic cloves, butter, and
   1 tablespoon of the chives to cauliflower and stir to combine.
   Serve, garnished with remaining 1 tablespoon chives.

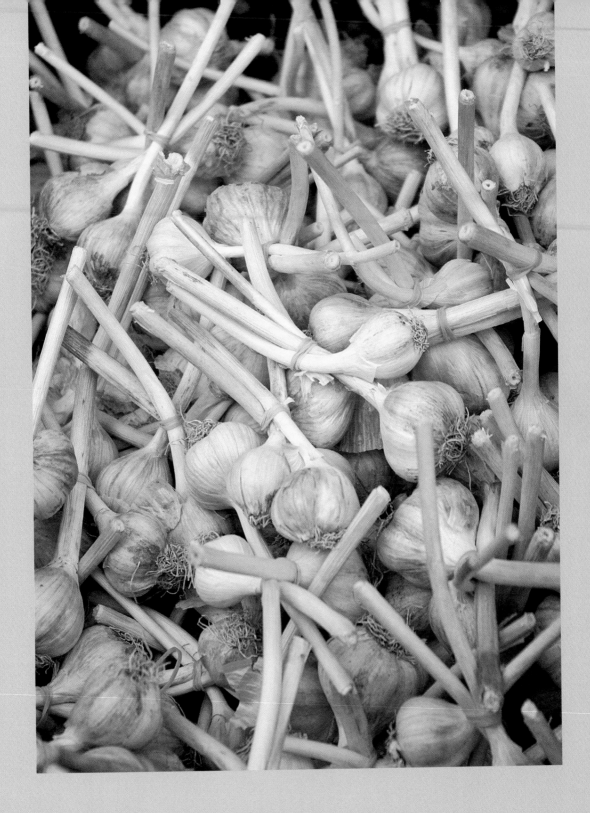

Spinach and Mushroom Lasagna

Substitute Gruyère or goat cheese for the mozzarella.

SERVES 4

9 (6-inch) Spinach Pancakes (pg. 30) ✓

Mushroom Layer:

1 tablespoon coconut or olive oil

1 small yellow onion, diced

4 garlic cloves, finely minced

1 pound medium-size button or
   cremini mushrooms, sliced

¼ cup finely chopped fresh basil

2 teaspoons finely chopped fresh thyme

Béchamel Layer:

3 tablespoons unsalted butter

3 tablespoons brown rice flour

3 cups whole milk or goat's milk, hot

1 teaspoon salt

½ teaspoon paprika

   Pinch of nutmeg

   Freshly ground black pepper

4 ounces mozzarella, shredded

2 ounces parmesan, grated

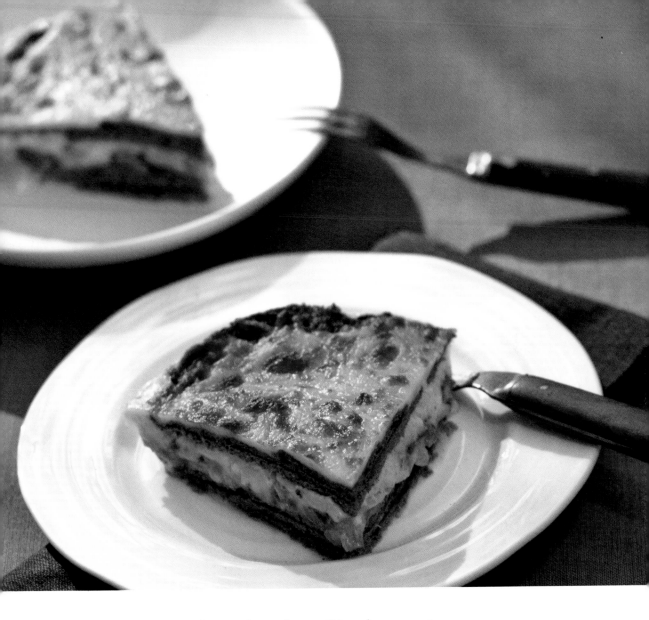

I. To make the mushroom layer, heat oil in a large sauté pan. Sauté onions until translucent, about 4 minutes. Add garlic and sauté for I minute. Add mushrooms and sauté until mushrooms have given up most of their liquid, about 5 minutes. Stir in basil and thyme. Remove from heat and set aside.

(continued)

2. To make the béchamel layer, place the butter and flour in a medium, heavy-bottomed saucepan over medium heat. Cook, stirring constantly, until mixture is smooth and thick. Turn heat to low and cook, stirring constantly, for 3 minutes, but do not allow roux to color. Remove from heat and add hot milk all at once, whisking vigorously to blend well.

3. Return to heat, stirring constantly with a whisk, and bring to a simmer. Let cook 3 minutes, until mixture is thick. Whisk in salt, paprika, nutmeg, and pepper. Remove from heat and set aside.

4. Preheat oven to 350° F.

5. To assemble: Spray a 10-inch round, deep pie or quiche dish with olive oil cooking spray. Spread about 1 cup of the béchamel on bottom of dish. Arrange 3 pancakes in a single layer over béchamel. Spread a third of the mushrooms and a third of the cheese on top. Repeat two more times the layers of béchamel pancakes, mushrooms, and cheese. Finish with the remaining pancakes and the remaining cheese.

6. Bake until bubbling and lightly browned on top, about 25 minutes. Allow to cool for about 20 minutes before serving.

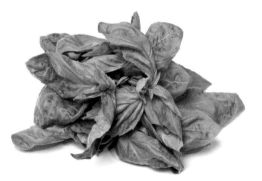

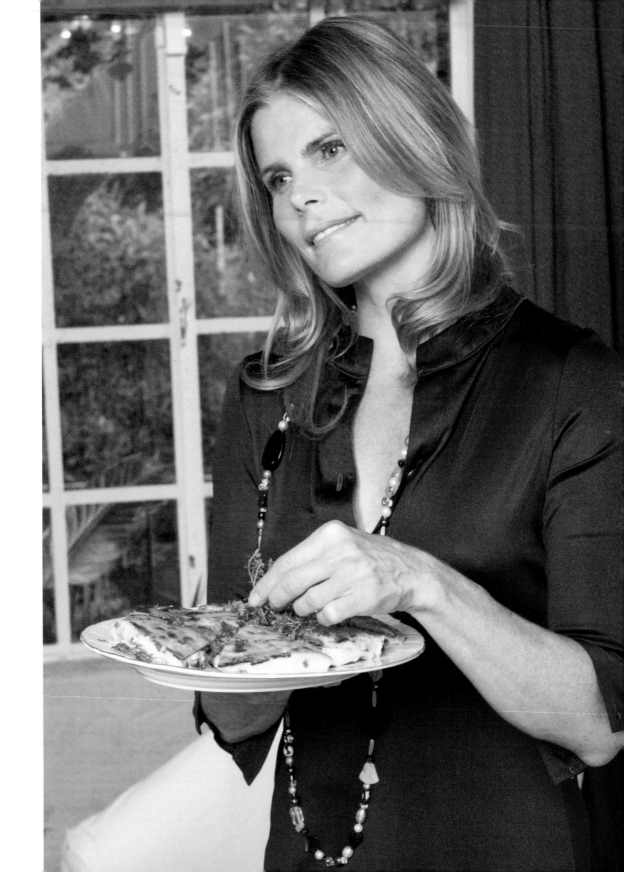

Pear Sorbet with Balsamic Port Syrup

If fresh vanilla beans aren't available, 1 teaspoon real vanilla extract can be added off-heat after the sauce has reduced. Crumble a Chocolate Blisscuit (pg. 38) on top for a crunchy garnish.

SERVES 6

- 1 cup plus 2 tablespoons Xylosweet
- ½ cup filtered water
- 6 medium-size organic pears, peeled and coarsely chopped
- 1 tablespoon lemon juice
- 1 cup balsamic vinegar
- 1 cup ruby port
- 1 vanilla bean, split, seeds scraped

1. Place ½ cup of the Xylosweet and all the water in a small saucepan over medium heat. Bring to a boil, reduce heat, and simmer for 2 to 3 minutes. Remove from heat and allow to cool completely.

2. Place pears, lemon juice, and 2 tablespoons of the Xylosweet in the work bowl of a food processor or blender. Add Xylosweet-water mixture and puree until smooth. Freeze mixture in an ice-cream maker according to manufacturer's recommendation. When frozen, pack into a freezer container and freeze until fully set.

3. Combine vinegar, port, split vanilla bean along with scraped seeds, and the remaining ½ cup Xylosweet in a heavy, medium saucepan. Bring to a boil, reduce heat to low, and simmer until sauce is thick and syrupy, about 30 minutes. Remove from heat and cool completely. Let cool to room temperature before serving.

4. To serve, scoop sorbet into individual serving bowls and top with a spoonful of sauce. Serve additional sauce on the side.

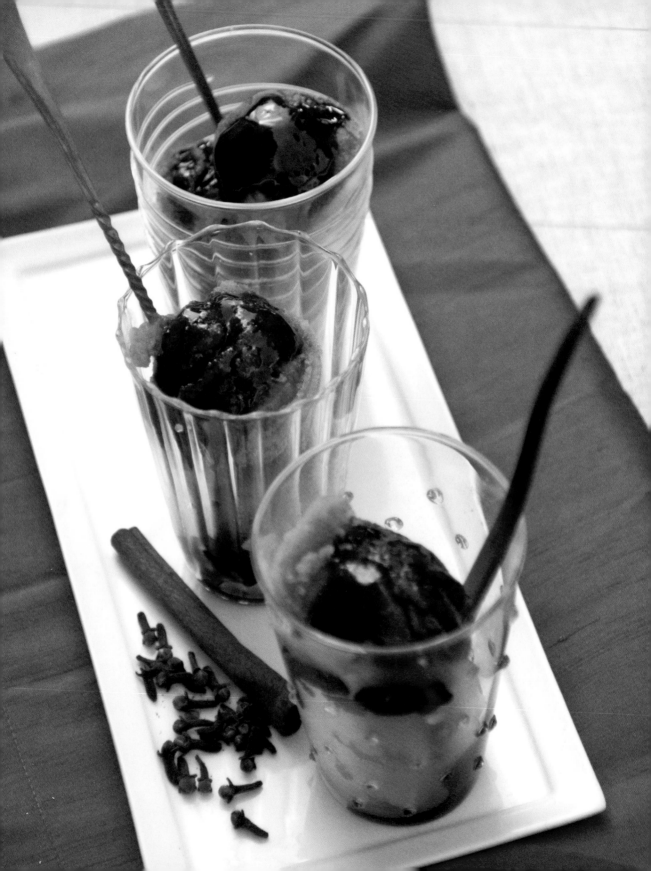

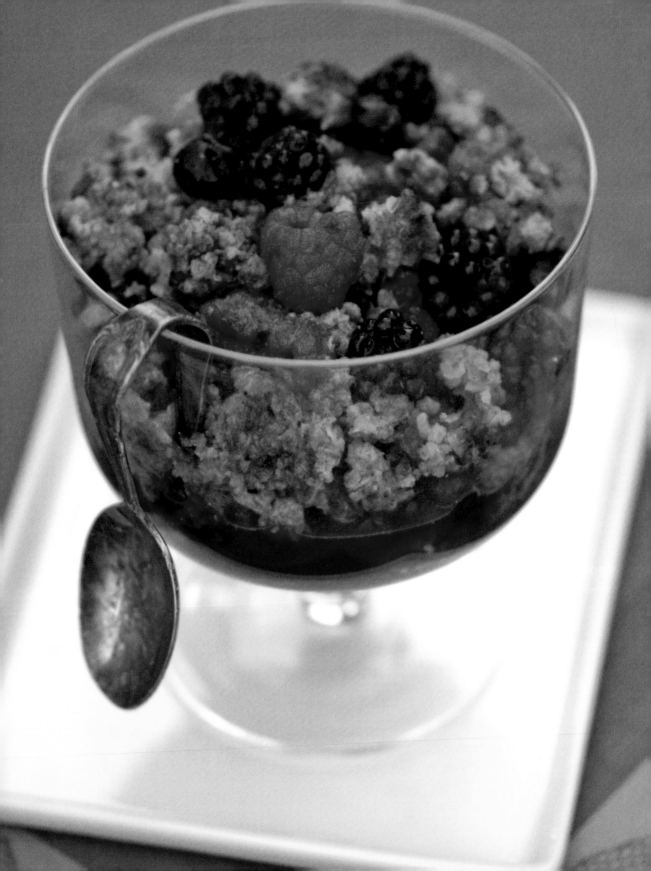

Berry Crisp

Coconut oil for greasing pan

8 cups mixed, seasonal organic berries

4 tablespoons Xylosweet — Brown sugar + Honey

3 tablespoons rice flour ~ Almond

1 cup rolled oats

½ teaspoon ground cinnamon

¼ teaspoon sea salt

½ cup unsalted butter, cut into small pieces and chilled

1. Preheat oven to 350°F.

2. Grease an 8- or 9-inch square baking dish with coconut oil.

3. Place berries in a large mixing bowl. (Larger fresh berries, such as strawberries, should be stemmed and sliced.) Add 2 tablespoons of the Xylosweet and 1 tablespoon of the flour, mixing gently to combine. Spoon into prepared baking dish and set aside.

4. Combine oats, the remaining 2 tablespoons Xylosweet, the remaining 2 tablespoons flour, cinnamon, and salt in a medium bowl, stirring to combine. Add butter pieces and blend into dry mixture using a fork or your fingers until it forms pea-size lumps, being careful not to overwork. Sprinkle mixture over the top of the berries.

5. Bake until berries are bubbling and topping begins to brown, 30 to 35 minutes. Allow to cool at least 15 minutes before serving.

If fresh berries are unavailable, substitute defrosted frozen organic berries.

Goat Cheese Tartlets

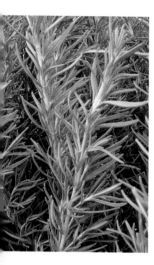

SERVES 6

  5 ounces goat cheese

  2 tablespoons heavy cream or goat's milk yogurt

  1 cup egg whites

⅛ teaspoon ground black pepper

  1 teaspoon fresh thyme leaves

    Coconut oil for greasing

12 sun-dried tomatoes, rehydrated in warm water for 20 minutes then patted dry

1. Preheat oven to 350°F.

2. In a mixing bowl combine goat cheese, cream, egg whites, pepper, and ½ teaspoon of the thyme, stirring until completely incorporated. Set aside.

3. Grease a mini muffin pan with coconut oil and place on a baking sheet. Press 1 sun-dried tomato into the bottom of each muffin compartment.

4. Spoon a small amount of goat cheese mixture over each sun-dried tomato, filling compartment about two-thirds of the way up. Garnish the top of each with a sprinkling of the remaining ½ teaspoon thyme leaves.

5. Bake for 20 to 30 minutes or until tartlets have risen and are golden brown on top.

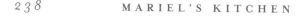

6. Let cool 10 minutes before running a small knife around the perimeter of each tartlet to ensure easy removal. Serve while still warm.

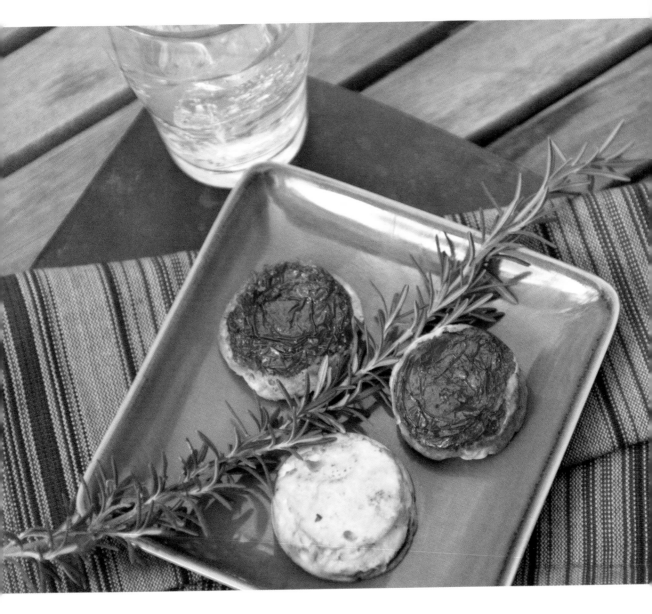

Baked Sweet Potato Sticks

2   sweet potatoes, peeled and cut into
    ¼ x ¼ x 2-inch sticks

2   tablespoons coconut or olive oil

½   tablespoon sea salt

1   teaspoon freshly ground black pepper

1. Preheat oven to 375°F.

2. Place sweet potato sticks in a large bowl and toss with the oil, salt, and pepper to coat.

3. Spread sweet potatoes in a single layer on the baking sheet. Bake for about 40 minutes or until the sweet potatoes are crisp on the outside and tender on the inside.

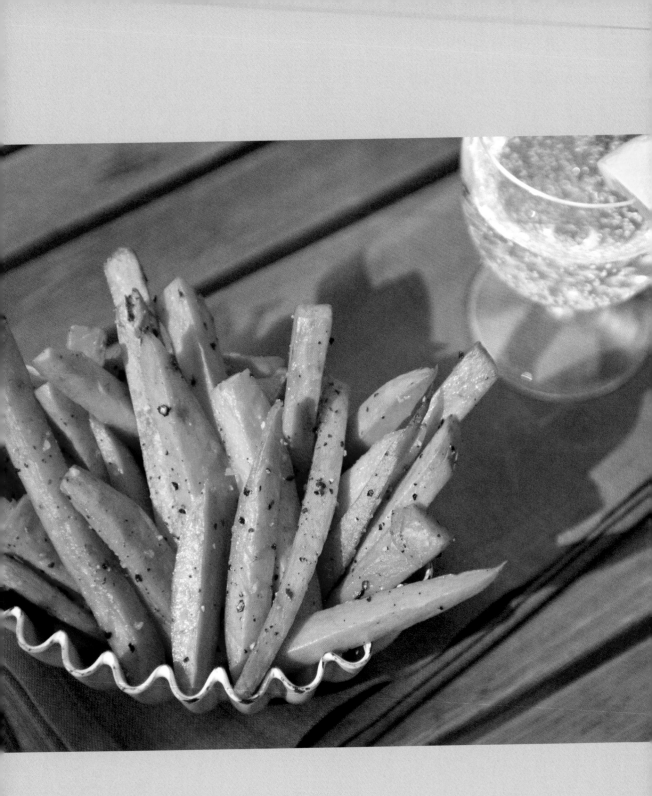

Faux Sangria

SERVES 6–8

¼ cup cubed apples, frozen

¼ cup cubed peaches, frozen

¼ cup cubed oranges, frozen

4 cups unsweetened pomegranate juice, chilled

3 tablespoons Xylosweet

3 cups sparkling water, chilled

1. Place all the cut fruit into a large punch bowl or pitcher.

2. Pour pomegranate juice over the fruit, add the Xylosweet, and stir until well combined.

3. Add the sparkling water and stir gently before serving.

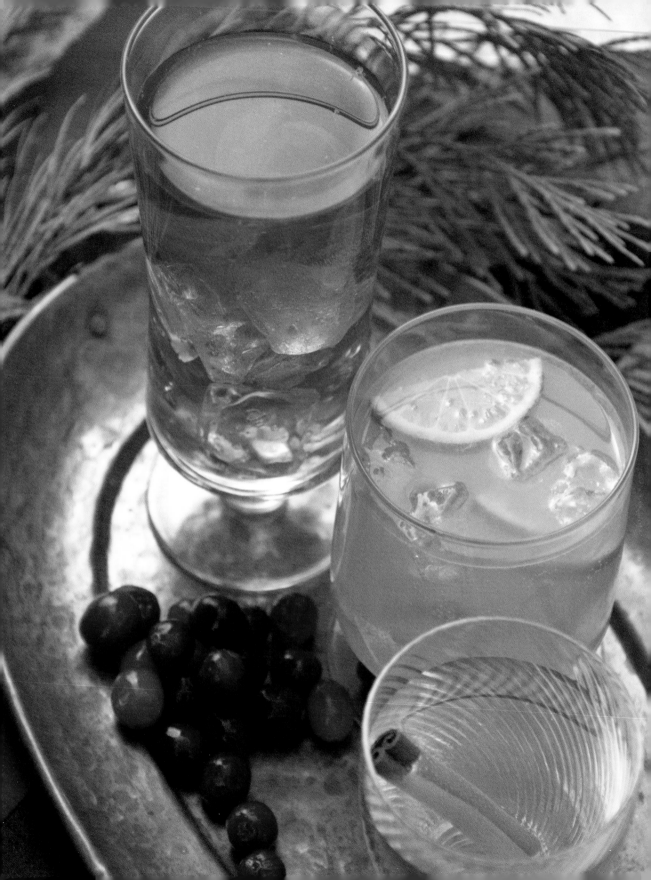

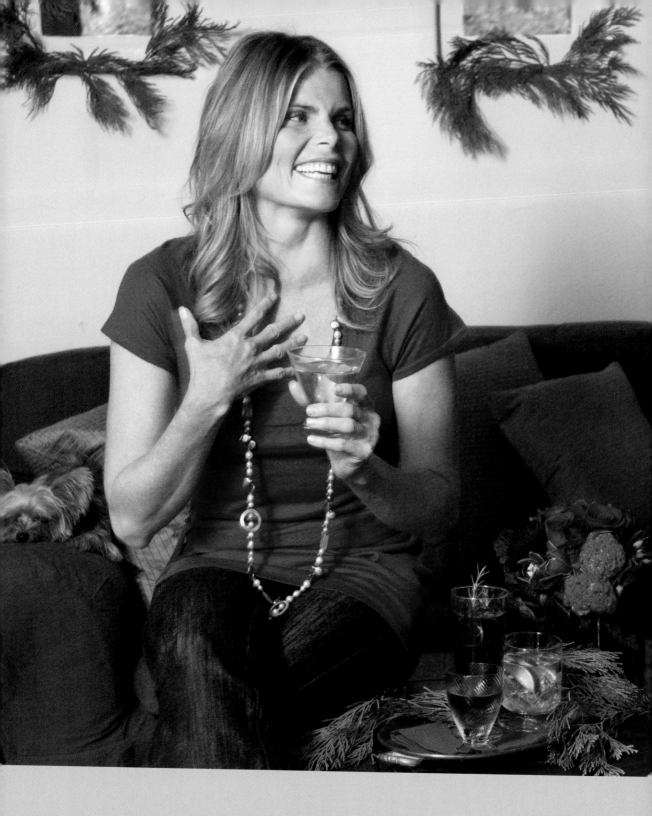

Faux Wine Spritzer

SERVES 6

4 cups unsweetened
   organic cranberry juice,
   chilled
2 cups sparkling water,
   chilled
½ cup fresh lime juice,
   chilled
¼ cup Xylosweet

1. Place all ingredients in a
   large punch bowl or pitcher
   filled with ice.
2. Stir to combine.

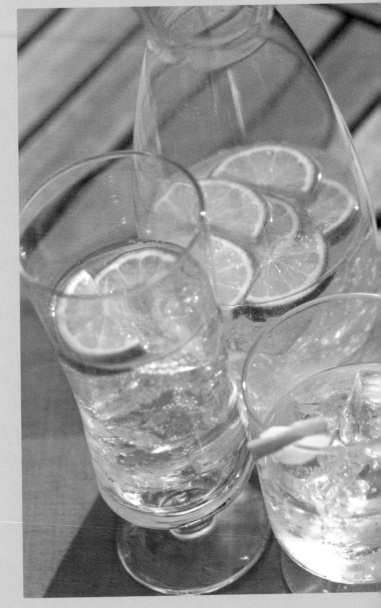

Hot Apple Cider

Using a channel knife or zester, cut curls of orange peel to add to this drink before squeezing the juice from the orange.

SERVES 6

  5 cups unfiltered apple juice

1 ½ cups freshly squeezed orange juice

  6 cinnamon sticks

12 whole cloves

1. Place all ingredients in a medium saucepan over medium-high heat. Bring to a boil, reduce heat, and simmer for 15 to 20 minutes.

2. Cover, remove from heat, and let steep for at least 20 minutes or as long as 1 hour.

3. Strain and serve. Can be served hot, warm, at room temperature, or chilled.

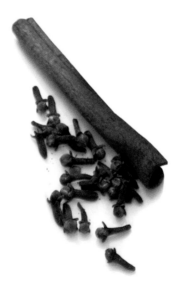

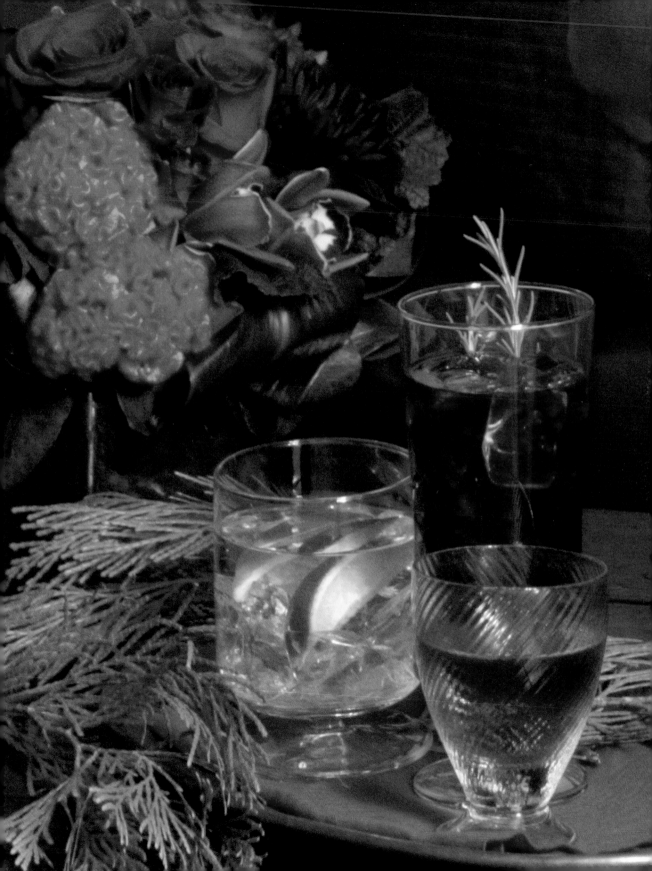

A Space to Love

For a kitchen to be the heart of the home, it should be a space you love to cook and eat in.
It doesn't require fancy décor. The room becomes memorable when you create an
atmosphere of health and joy.

1 Natural light **is a precious resource in the kitchen (and it's free!). Just as the world outside flourishes and grows** when bathed in the sun's energy, so do we. Position the table where you eat to catch what daylight you can, especially in winter; it is healing, nourishing, and adds to the eating experience. Make sure your kitchen lighting at night is bright and warm for cooking— and ideally, can be dimmed for eating.

2 If you have no natural light source available, bring the outside in through other means. **Plants and indoor trees, herb containers, tabletop fountains or even aquariums fill the area with nature.**

3 Take the space beyond just functional. **Make it comfortable. Do you have somewhere to sit as your stew** simmers? Do your friends have a place to relax while you cook? Small touches like adding cushions to stools or bringing in an armchair will make the kitchen a room to live in, not just a place to do daily tasks.

4 Make even kitchen table lunches a little sacred. **I set each place with cutlery, a cloth napkin, a water glass,** and light a candle. It makes the act of eating mindful, not mindless; I notice what I eat and enjoy it more, and these details needn't add more time to the prep.

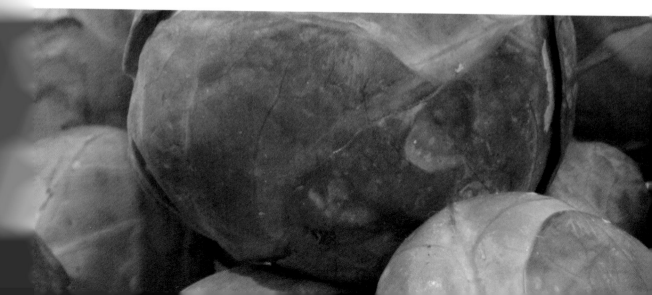

5 In winter, bring greenery inside. I place a few branches of pine in the center of the table, on a windowsill or in the hearth, throughout the season, not just at Christmas. The smell and sense of comfort it brings to the room is amazing. I also love to bring in rosemary from my pots in the garden and let it dry hanging from cupboard knobs; it provides instant winter aromatherapy.

6 Let simple weekday suppers soothe your senses. With some candles, some classical music (proven to help digestion—I like Bach's Concerto #5) and full license to wear your coziest slippers, even soup and salad become a little moment of "loving you." Kids or teenagers will probably run to their rooms. Let them! If you have a fireplace somewhere in the home, camp out by it and make dinner a picnic. Eating can and should be both healthy and sensual.

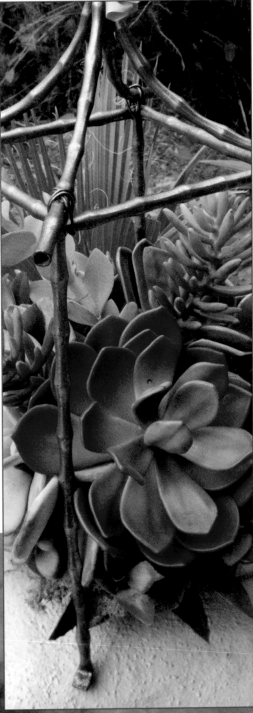

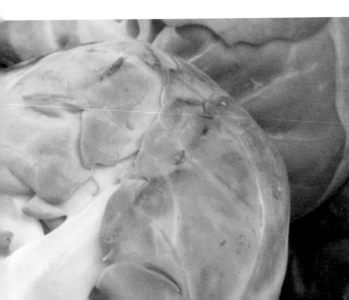

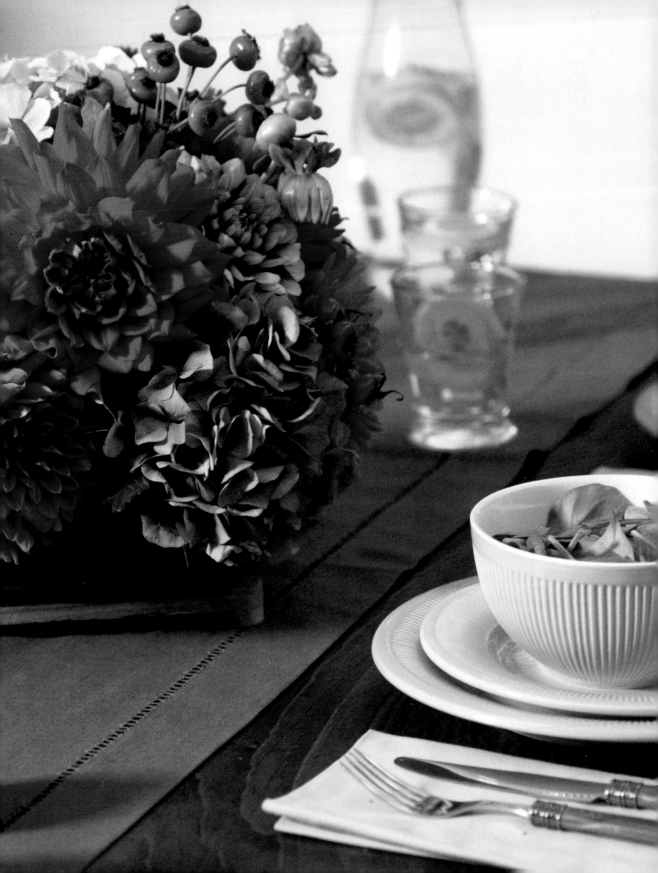

Some Final Thoughts:
Finding the Sacred in Food

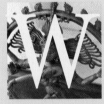e all have a relationship to food that is at once joyous and infuriating. Food is a basic essential; we can't get away from it. We have to eat to survive and thrive. It appears, in this country especially, that we've turned desperate around food, through over indulgence. This may seem contradictory, yet let me explain. We love to eat because we love the feeling that food gives us. It is nurturing, it is grounding. Often, however, that feeling is a replacement for our sense of well-being and love. By nature, humans want more love—that's all anybody really wants—so we turn to food to get a sense of self. It's easier that way, because it has no person attached to it, judging us or finding reasons we shouldn't be loved. So we eat more, because if love is what we desire, we certainly want more of it. We anthropomorphize food,

making it our friend, our lover, our partner, our therapist. This takes away the need to look at the deeper issues of why we feel unloved.

Food is such a beautiful part of our lives. I want to invite people and myself to gracefully find a way to turn food into a valued ceremony that enhances our lives on every level. Instead of making food a person, I would like to make food another essence of myself. Food becomes that which expresses my delicacy as a woman and as a being who cares for herself.

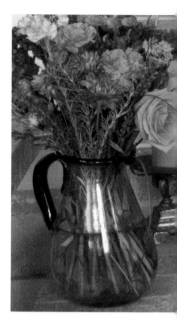

When food is overindulged in, it takes on qualities of a master and slave. Food becomes the master and the eater becomes its slave. With that, there comes the constant need to please. You become split within yourself. Instead of being true to your essence and your nature, you serve your outer self, the one ruled by food. If food can come down from the realm of regal master and become our inner essence, everyone benefits. We slow down, eat with conscious awareness of how we chew, how we set a table, what we prepare for the enhancement of our essence. If food becomes our artistic expression, then we all become very careful in the implementation of our gift. Our making of nourishment becomes the act with which we create something that, like a sand mandala that gets blown out of existence by the wind, is not permanently in sight but is constant in our being.

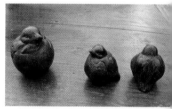

Still, the energy that was put into the food stays with us and moves into our cells, into our sense of self. It becomes the essence of us. It can be healing when we have made it from love instead of using it as the outer expression of a love that is hollow and perhaps not real love at all.

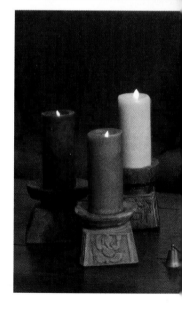

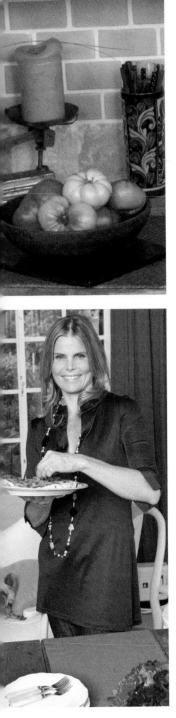

Real food is like real love; it is born of the earth. It grows like some kind of miracle that we have come to take for granted. Yet the journey I am on right now is to remember where my food has come from, the journey that it has taken from field to plate. This is not woo woo stuff! This is awareness of life and how we inhabit the planet. This is about all people becoming themselves deeply, caring for their world by caring for themselves. To some extent, we make food and try new recipes to satisfy the needs of our bodies and families, and sometimes to impress the outside world. But we can also see it as developing our inner world, using the deliberate act of choosing and cooking food as a very basic practice of becoming more authentic. When we step back, become quiet, and consider that food may come from something greater than ourselves, however we want to picture that, whether as Nature, Spirit, Source, Gaia, or God, our awareness shifts. Food consciousness, I believe, is a foundation of our spiritual life.

Throughout history, in all sacred places, the ritual of food has a profound place in the connection to the spirit. Whether in the preparation, the sacrament, the blessing, the intent, or the symbolism, cooking is understood to be a ritual of connection and devotion. Done consciously, it becomes sacred to the development of your sense of self and your connection to your bigger self, that part of you that is already perfect. Care for your inner environment by being aware of your participation in the outer environment, that place the sustenance comes from, and you feel a deeper connection to yourself as a unique expression of the divine.

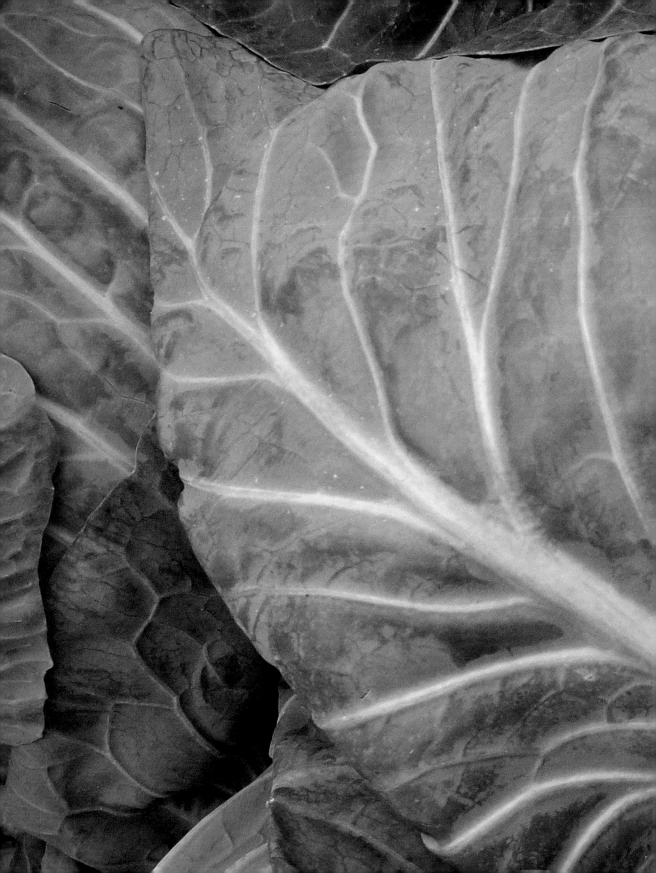

Resources

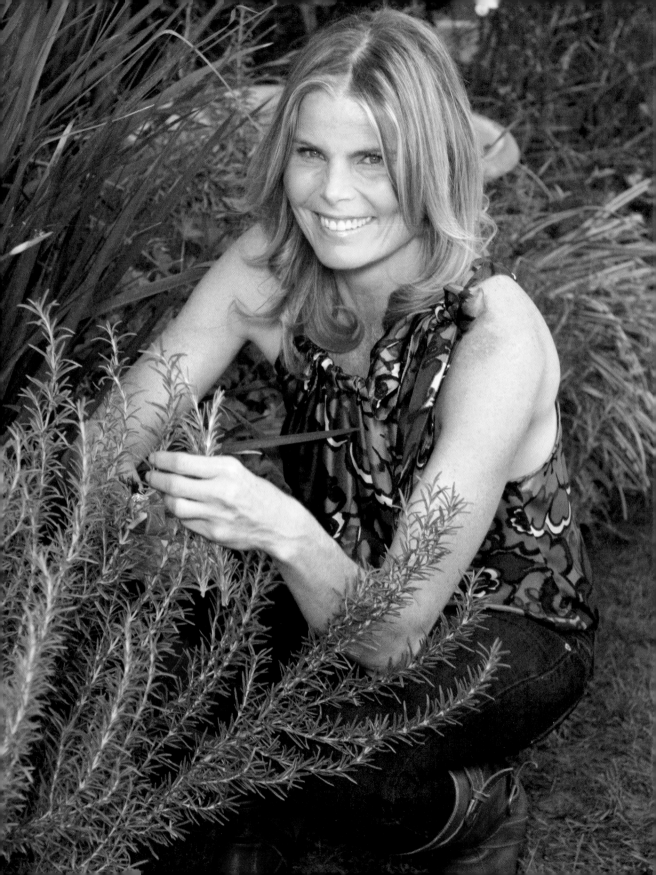

Green Pages

Here are some of the products, people, and information sources that have helped me create a simple, seasonal, and sustainable kitchen.

INGREDIENTS

Most of the ingredients featured in the Pantry Essentials section have Web sites that provide reams of information about the health benefits of their products. You can become a food expert simply by stocking your cupboards. Read and enjoy!

Organic extra virgin coconut oil & hemp protein powder

Nutiva, www.nutiva.com. You may want to try Nutiva's hemp protein powder for shakes—this is especially useful if you are vegan and don't want to eat whey (dairy) protein. The cold-pressed hemp oil is good on salads and vegetables, and another good source of healthy essential fats.

Whey protein
Jay Robb, www.jayrobb.com.

Xylosweet & SweetLeaf Stevia
Xlear, www.xlear.com, and SweetLeaf Sweetener, www.sweetleaf.com.

Flours
Bob's Red Mill, www.bobsredmill .com, and Authentic Foods, www .authenticfoods.com. The latter also has xanthan gum.

Ume plum vinegar
Eden Organic, www.edenfoods.com.

Herbs
AeroGarden, www.aerogarden.com. You can get these small, streamlined indoor herb-growing units to supply your kitchen with fresh herbs even in the February chill. Spices are best bought from local stores; a food co-op or Indian food store is a good source when you are buying numerous kinds.

Himalayan salt
Himalayan Living Salt, www.himala yanlivingsalt.com. One of the earth's natural health wonders, this can also be used therapeutically for detox baths.

Quinoa
There are many brands and bulk-aisle options of quinoa available. I like Alter Eco Fair Trade, www .alterecopacific.com, for its fair-trade products from Bolivia (which include chocolate and teas).

Teas
Rishi Tea, www.rishi-tea.com, and SerendipiTea, www.serendipitea.com, are two of my favorite sources. The famous New York store Takashimaya, www.takashimaya-ny.com, has exquisite Japanese blends.

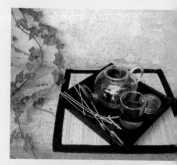

Some more foods and drinks to try:

I avoid bottled water for daily use, but I do use two products strategically because they support health in powerful ways.

O2Cool Oxygen Water
www.hiosilver.com, has a high level of oxygen for extra energy as well as high magnesium, a critical nutrient that most of us are severely lacking today. Noah's water, www.noahs7up .com, is another great source of magnesium.

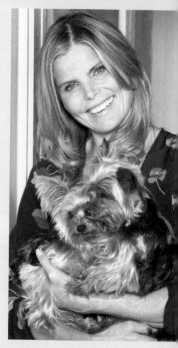

Nativas naturals

www.nativasnaturals.com, will blow you away with the exciting options for adding superfood powders to your breakfast smoothies and has energizing raw cacao and dried Amazon fruits for snacks.

O.N.E.

www.onenaturalexperience.com, is one of many new kinds of coconut water on the market.

Three Dog Bakery

www.threedog.com, makes fantastic "real food" dog chow for your most loyal furry friend.

PRODUCTS AND GADGETS FOR YOUR KITCHEN

Gaiam

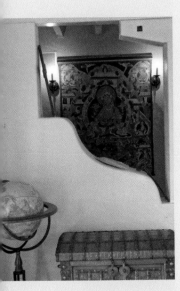

www.gaiam.com, is my trusted source for green cleaning products and household items that help simplify sustainable living, shopping, and more. My favorite find is one of their most affordable—the countertop bag dryer. I use the To-Go Ware food tin for taking meals on the road. I also use the stainless steel water bottles and compost crock, and stock up on organic cotton kitchen cloths. Gaiam is a conscious company that has done its research on every product. Together we also put out the *Yoga Now* DVDs that I make with my friend Rodney Yee.

✓ Target

www.target.com, makes the processes of cooking and entertaining easier by offering affordable cookware and appliances (like a waffle maker for my winter breakfast recipe). They are introducing more eco-friendly items and will be carrying my new line of healthy foods, also called Mariel's Kitchen—no prizes for guessing the first product. Blisscuits! I hope you will give them a try and let me know your thoughts via my Web site, listed at the end of this section.

✓ Oxygen Ozone

www.oxygenozone.com, has great nine-stage water filters that fit under the sink and remove every trace of harmful dirt, chemical and, as we're now discovering, prescription-drug residue, from city-supplied H_2O.

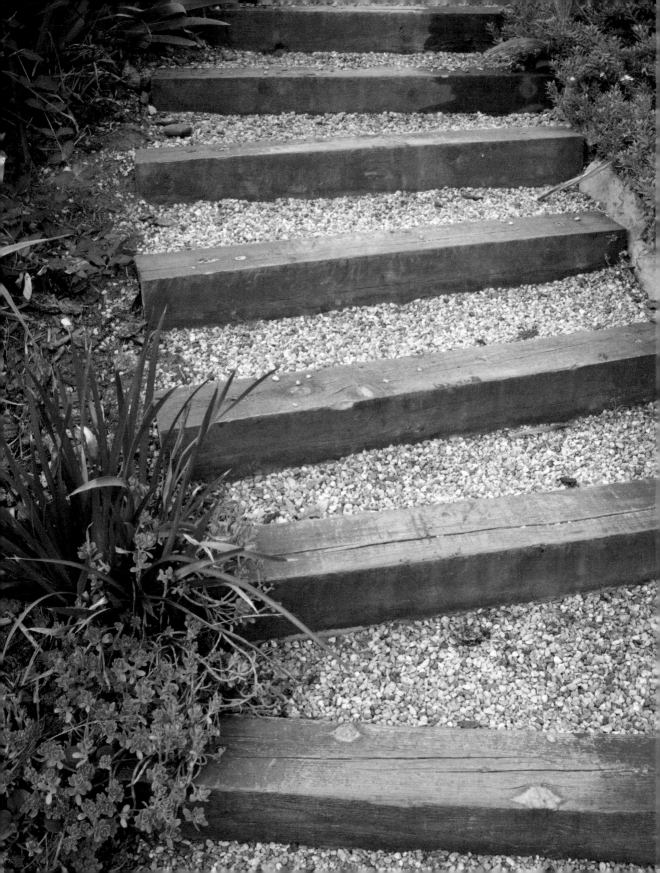

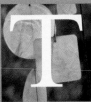anks for taking this journey through food with me. Please visit my blog, www.marielhemingway.org/blog, for more of my discoveries. You can write me your experiences of cooking my recipes—and share some of your own ideas for simple and satisfying meals. I would love to hear from you!

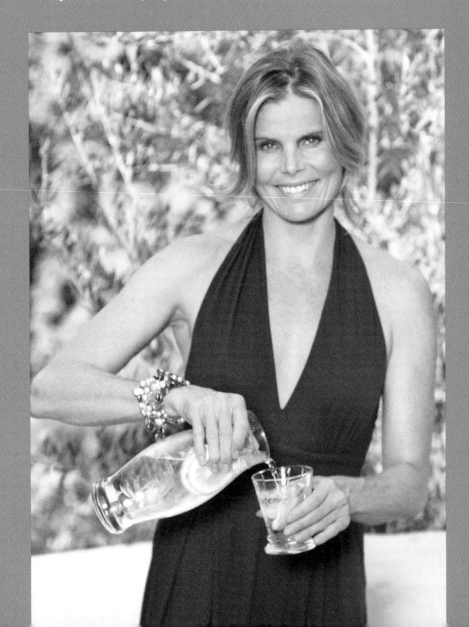

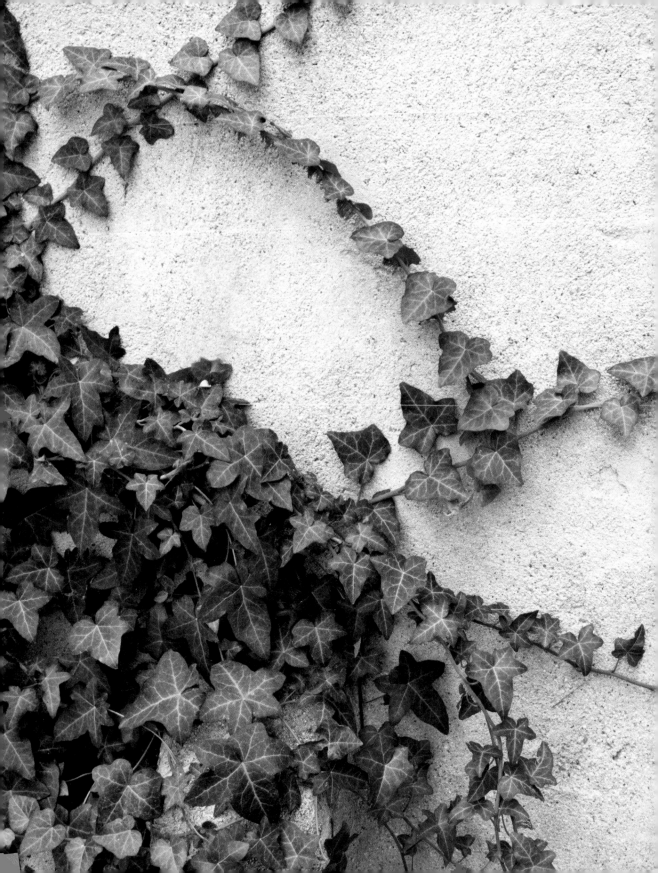

Acknowledgments

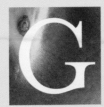ood, healthful cooking doesn't happen without a great team. From the farmers to the chefs, everyone involved work together to create great meals for our tables. And so the same can be said for making a great cookbook. I had such a fun time spending a few weeks in my home with my team to photograph and cook all the delicious recipes you see in this book. Everyone did an exceptional job in bringing my idea of good, organic meals to your tables.

I'd like to thank Jeff Katz, and his crew Andrew Strauss and Stuart Gow, for their beautiful photographs. And Denise Vivaldo and Cindie Flannigan of FoodFanatics, who helped me refine my recipes so that they can be easily prepared and tastier than ever. Thank you also to Jennifer Park, Sarah Bush, Travis Witten, Matt Armendariz, and Karine Beaudry for their help with our food preparations. We couldn't have done it without you! A special thanks to my friends Golriz Moeini and Nico Guilis for assisting me during the photo shoot—you thought of everything—and to Magnolia boutique for their wonderful wardrobe collections. Thank you also to art director, Beth Tondreau, for her management and coordination during the photo sessions and her beautiful designs and layouts.

And finally, I'd like to thank Amely Greeven, my editor, Gideon Weil, and the HarperOne team, Terri Leonard, Jan Baumer, and Carolyn Allison-Holland for helping me bring my vision of good healthful living from my kitchen to yours.

Happy cooking,

Mariel

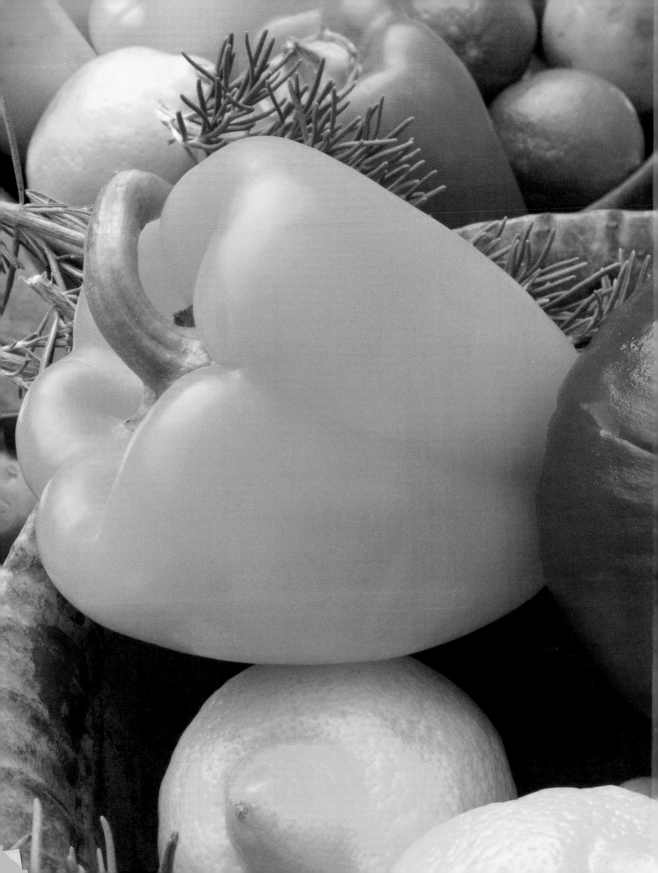